Consuming

Consuming Health explores the diverse meanings and applications of the term 'consumer' in the field of health care and assesses the implications for policy-making, health care delivery and experiences of health care. Combining social and critical perspectives with empirical examples, it focuses on contemporary issues and areas of practice including:

- young people, drug use and consumption of health;
- consumerism in mental health care;
- health consumer groups and the national policy process;
- care in the hospital and the community;
- the language of consumerism and its use.

With contributions from well-known and innovative researchers and practitioners, this is a book that challenges assumptions. At the same time, it does not assume prior knowledge of key issues and perspectives but is student-friendly, providing an all-round view of consumerism as applied to health care.

Saras Henderson is a Senior Lecturer in the School of Nursing and Midwifery, Curtin University of Technology, Perth, Western Australia. **Alan Petersen** is a Professor in Sociology of Health and Illness in the Department of Sociology, University of Plymouth, UK.

Consuming Health

The commodification
of health care

Edited by Saras Henderson
and Alan Petersen

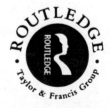

London and New York

First published 2002
by Routledge
11 New Fetter Lane, London EC4P 4EE

Simultaneously published in the USA and Canada
by Routledge
29 West 35th Street, New York, NY 10001

Routledge is an imprint of the Taylor & Francis Group

British Library Cataloguing in Publication Data
A catalogue record for this book is available from the British
Library

Library of Congress Cataloging in Publication Data
Consuming health : the commodification of health care / edited by
Saras Henderson and Alan Petersen.
Includes bibliographical references and index.
1. Social medicine. 2. Medical care–Social aspects. 3. Consumers.
I. Henderson, Saras, 1950– II. Petersen, Alan R., Ph. D.

RA418 .C672 2001
362.1'042–dc21
                                                    200141822

ISBN 0–415–25948–7 (hbk)
ISBN 0–415–25949–5 (pbk)

Contents

Contributors

Judith Allsop is a Research Professor in Health Policy at De Montfort University, Leicester and co-director of the Health Policy Research Unit. She is also an emeritus professor at South Bank University, London.

Rob Baggott is Professor of Public Policy and Director of the Health Policy Research Unit at De Montfort University.

Robin Bunton is Reader in Social Policy in the School of Human Studies at the University of Teesside, UK.

Alexander Clark is a researcher in the Department of Public Health, Glasgow University, Scotland.

Michael Clinton is Professor of the School of Public Health, Curtin University of Technology, Perth, Western Australia.

Paul Crawshaw is a researcher and teaches sociology in the school of Social Sciences at the University of Teeside, UK.

Elizabeth Ettorre is Professor of Sociology, Department of Sociology, University of Plymouth, UK.

Arthur W. Frank is Professor of Sociology at the University of Calgary in Canada.

Susan Hansen is a PhD candidate at the School of Psychology, Murdoch University, and a research officer at the Eastern Perth Public and Community Health Unit.

Mike Hazelton is Professor of Mental Health Nursing, Faculty of Nursing, the University of Newcastle, New South Wales, Australia.

Saras Henderson is Senior Lecturer in Nursing, School of Nursing and Midwifery at Curtin University of Technology in Perth, Western Australia.

Rob Irvine is a Lecturer in the Department of Sociology and Anthropology, University of Newcastle, New South Wales, Australia.

Kathryn Jones is the full-time ESRC research fellow on the Health Consumer Groups project, at De Montfort University, Leicester, UK.

Renata Kokanovic is a sociologist working at Eastern Perth Public and Community Health Unit (EPP & CHU), Western Australia in the mental health promotion programme and conducting research in ethnicity, mental health and illness.

Steven Miles is Principal Lecturer in Sociology, Department of Sociology, University of Plymouth, UK.

Alan Petersen is Professor in Sociology of Health and Illness, Department of Sociology, University of Plymouth, UK.

Anthony Pryce is Reader in Sexual Health, Department of Applied Psychosocial Sciences, City University, St Bartholomew School, London, UK.

Margaret Reid is Reader in the Department of Public Health, Glasgow University, Scotland.

Pekka Sulkunen is Professor, Department of Sociology, University of Helsinki, Finland.

Acknowledgements

We would like to thank all those who agreed to contribute to this project and who willingly agreed to our demands for revisions. We are grateful to Edwina Welham who commissioned this book and Michelle Bacca who assisted in answering our queries. We acknowledge the support of our respective universities, the Curtin University of Technology and Murdoch University, which allowed us the time and resources necessary to write and to compile the collection. Finally, we are grateful to our partners, Bernard Smith and Ros Porter, whose love and support sustained us throughout the book's long maturation period.

Introduction

Consumerism in health care

Saras Henderson and Alan Petersen

Recent dramatic changes in health care in many contemporary societies, involving the deregulation and privatization of services and an emphasis on cost-effectiveness, 'user-pays', 'self-care', 'community-based care', and so on, pose important challenges for policy-makers, health care workers and recipients of health care. Increasingly, health is viewed as a 'commodity' and individuals are defined as health care 'consumers'. The language of consumerism has become pervasive in health care, reflecting a changed relationship between citizens and the state from that which characterized many, if not most, liberal democratic societies in the past. The notion that the state should care for the health of its citizens, long seen as a fundamental principle of welfare states, is increasingly replaced by the expectation that citizens should play a more active role in caring for themselves as 'clients' or 'consumers'. The view that citizens *should* be consumers of health and health care, and that they *do* indeed conduct themselves as such, however, is by no means uncontentious or uncontested. This book explores the diverse and often complex meanings and applications of the term 'consumer' in the arena of health care and assesses the implications for policy-making, health care delivery and people's experiences of health care. It asks, who are the assumed 'consumers' of health care policy and practice, and what exactly is it that they are 'consuming'? How relevant is the consumerism model in the field of health care? Is it valid and useful to view health and health care as 'commodities'? What are the social, political and ethical implications of the consumerism in health care? How does the deployment of the philosophy and language of consumerism in the health care field affect people's experience of illness and the nature and quality of care? And, how might the language and practices of consumerism be used to advance the interests of those who are ill, and promote change in health care systems?

Recent efforts to apply the consumerism model in health care would seem to reflect a more general tendency towards consumerism in social life, as observed in many contemporary societies. However, while the subject of consumption as an aspect of contemporary culture has been of growing interest to many scholars, there has been relatively little analysis of consumption and consumerism as applied specifically to health and health care. Much work thus far has been concerned with describing the character-istics and practices of 'consumer society', a term popularized by Jean Baudrillard in his now famous *The Consumer Society*, first published in 1970 and released in its English translation in 1998. As Baudrillard (1998: 80) has argued, in modern societies consumption has become institutional-ized, not as a right or pleasure, but as a *duty* of the citizen. Further, people consume not only goods, but also human services and therefore human rela-tionships. Indeed, virtually everything becomes an object of consumption. Consumption has become a way of thinking and a way of life, and provides the very basis for our concept of self, or identity. In a culture saturated by the mass media, the symbolic realm itself is 'consumable'; that which we consume is not so much what is signified by the message, but the message itself (1998: 122–3). Others, building on this work, have subsequently explored the body as a site and object of consumption (Falk 1994; Featherstone 1991), the production of the consuming self and of individual desire (Bauman 1998; Sulkunen *et al.* 1997), and the contexts and rituals of consumption (Urry 1995; Corrigan 1997; Miles 1998). While research has been diverse, topics such as the shopping experience, the processes and impacts of advertising, and the consumer practices of particular groups (e.g. youth) have figured prominently in the recent literature. Clearly, a signifi-cant amount of this work pertains to the consumption of goods rather than of services and to sites where conditions of 'perfect' competition in a 'free market' are seen to prevail. (See, for example, the recent collections by Lee (2000) and Miller (2001).) In the arena of health care, however, the opera-tions of the market have been less evident or are more contentious, and the state has tended to play an interventionist role by way of protecting what have been seen to be entitlements or rights, via citizens' charters, for example. With recent rapid changes in the philosophies and practices of health and welfare, and the erosion of many established rights, there needs to be a thoroughgoing assessment of the impact of consumerism on health and health care, and of the implications for those who are defined as the 'consumers'.

One important focus of this book is the conception of self that has accompanied the shift from 'welfarist' to 'neo-liberal' politics in health care. As scholars who are concerned with issues of governance have emphasized, in the post-welfare era, rule is premised increasingly on the concept of the active subject or citizen (e.g. Barry *et al.* 1996; Burchell *et al.* 1991; Rose 1999). Writers have noted a change in terminology to describe the subjects of health care – from 'patient' to 'client' or 'consumer' – corresponding with the emergence of this new active citizenship. Whereas the former term suggests passivity and diminished capacity for independent decision-making, the latter implies a capacity for independent decision-making, and a readiness to put information to use (Brock 1995: 158–9). Consumerism is often presented in terms of personal empowerment and freedom of choice. However, behind the rhetoric of 'freedom of choice', 'right to know', and 'entitlement to participate', that has recently come to dominate discussions in health care, lie compulsions surrounding the exercise of choice and an array of predefined and limited options for action. The 'good consumer' of health care is compelled to make choices, to exhibit appropriate 'information-seeking' behaviour, and to behave in certain prescribed ways (consulting 'relevant' expertise, taking the 'right' medicine, engaging in personal risk management, and so on). As a number of the contributors to this book make clear, however, one can question the extent to which this ideal of rational consumer behaviour accords with the reality of people's everyday lives. When people are affected by conditions that involve stigmatization – such as mental illness and sexual diseases – they may be reluctant, or unable, to seek help in the prescribed ways or may not engage with services in predictable, ideal 'rational' ways. (See Chapters 7 and 9.) Further, the depiction of health care services in terms of the consumer model, evident in the use of terms such as 'provider' and 'purchaser' (e.g. the so-called purchaser–provider split of the UK's NHS), can be questioned on a number of grounds (Hugman 1994: 216; Shackley and Ryan 1994). In a highly diverse society, marked by differences of class, ethnicity, gender, and so on, it needs to be asked how relevant this model is, and whether the services that are provided or 'sold' are necessarily what users, or potential users, require. Cross-cultural differences in conceptions of health and illness, and differences in access to resources such as education and work, will affect definitions of need, 'information-seeking' behaviour, and propensity to use services.

Despite the relative neglect of the analysis of consumerism in health care, scholars researching in this area have increasingly acknowledged the importance of consumerist trends, with some recent work addressing one or more aspects of consumption in particular domains of health care practice. Hogg, for example, has drawn attention to the limits of the notion of the patient as consumer in a context in which it is often unclear whether the consumer is the patient or the carer, and in which service users cannot learn from experience and have restricted knowledge and choice. As Hogg (1999: 169–71) observes, while individual choice and freedom might be important values, they may shift the focus away from the community and collective approaches to participation that are necessary to advance the health and well-being of the population as a whole. Others have noted that, in consumer culture, 'need' and 'choice' are always already constrained by the prevailing symbolic and value systems, which attach certain meaning and significance to certain behaviours and patterns of consumption (Frank 2000; Grace 1991; 1994). Thus, the consumption of particular health-related goods and services is shaped not simply by perceived health benefits (improved health), but also by their associations with particular images, lifestyles, and tastes. One of the major limitations with recent health promotion strategies has been the failure to acknowledge the role of culture in shaping tastes and preferences. In a context in which health, consumption, and identity are increasingly intertwined, it is naïve to believe that the actions of individuals are shaped solely by considerations of 'health' (Bunton and Burrows 1995). The adoption of the marketing approach in health promotion, which implies a neat dualistic distinction between the 'consumers' who have needs, wants, and desires, and the service providers or marketeers, who have plans, targets, and goals, denies the relations of power and knowledge existing between 'consumers' and providers. It implies that the former have needs or lacks, which can be satisfied simply through the provision, purchase, and consumption of goods and services (Grace 1991: 334–5). Finally, the findings of some recent empirical work question whether people think of themselves or act as consumers. When communicating with doctors, for instance, patients often do not exhibit information-seeking behaviour but rather prefer doctors to take on the responsibility for decision-making (Shackley and Ryan 1994: 532–6; Lupton *et al.* 1991). Also, lay people may adopt both 'consumerist' and 'passive patient' roles at the same time, or variously, depending on the context (Lupton 1997). Taken as a whole, this recent work, which draws on the insights offered by writers such as Baudrillard, Bourdieu, and Foucault, has helped to recast thinking about the status and autonomy of the 'health consumer'. What is taken to be the autonomous rational 'consumer' of health care can be seen to be largely an artefact of culture, expertise, and the health-marketing system (see, e.g., Grace 1994).

Although, clearly, they are socially and historically constructed, the identity label 'the consumer' and the language of consumerism have proved useful to numerous groups in their efforts to make visible their claims of health disadvantage and to protect and advance their interests. The strategic use of identity labels, or so-called 'strategic essentialism', where groups assume a cohesive identity for specific political purposes, has been shown to be effective in feminist struggles and in advancing the position of minority and disadvantaged groups (see Spivak 1993). Given its importance as a basis for identity in late modern societies, 'consumption' provides a powerful means for protecting or (re)claiming citizenship rights and for mobilizing to affect longer term change. Employing mechanisms such as the Patient's (or Citizen's) Charter, which specify rights (and responsibilities), consumer protection legislation, and the like, citizen-consumers have been able to organize to protect not only their own interests but the interests of those who are relatively disadvantaged and disempowered (e.g. mentally ill people). Thus, consumerism has a complex 'double-edged' character by providing (a) the basis for regulation over bodies and lives and obscuring, through its focus on the individual consumer, the need for social change; and (b) an identity label and language for (re)claiming rights for disadvantaged groups. A number of the chapters in this book explore these paradoxes of consumerism, focusing on the ways in which consumer communities have used, or may use, the language of consumerism to advance health.

In what follows, we make no claim to comprehensiveness in our presentation of topics, perspectives, and practice-settings. Comprehensiveness is not possible since consumerism is likely to manifest somewhat differently in different contexts and at different times. The philosophy of consumerism, the practices of consumption, and the extent of the commodification of health and health care are likely to vary considerably between countries, and even within health care systems, as will the meanings of the terms used to describe these phenomena. For example, notions of 'consumer choice' differ between the UK and France, which is based on universal health insurance with independent and public providers, and enshrines patients' rights to choose their doctor, and gives doctors the freedom to prescribe and practise where they wish (see Hogg 1999: 170). Similarly, the US health care system, which is highly deregulated and heavily dependent on both the private health sector and contributions of private health insurance, will entail different consumer imperatives from those operating in the more socialized systems of Europe and Australia. Consequently, we would caution against generalizing from the conclusions arising from the following accounts to other contexts of health and health care. However, as will become evident, the chapters present certain recurring themes and criticisms in relation to the use of these terms and the phenomena they purport to describe. Contributors have been invited to contribute to the book on the basis of their standing in the field and their known research interests, their potential to offer novel insights, and their ability to write in an accessible style. Our collection includes scholars based in the UK, Canada, Finland, and Australia. Our aims have been (a) to stimulate debate on a topic that, although clearly in need of systematic and critical analysis, has been largely neglected in the scholarly literature, (b) to expose and challenge the rhetoric of consumerism, and (c) to provide a text for teaching and the foundation for further research. In some sense, and to some extent, we are all positioned as 'consumers' of health and health care; therefore, we not only have experiences as 'consumers', but have the ability to use the language of consumerism in a strategic manner to affect change. It is our belief that effective change – successful 'treatment' – always presupposes an accurate 'diagnosis'. With this in mind, we would like to invite you to join us in an effort to diagnose consumerism as it operates in contemporary health and health care, so that we may better understand its implications – its benefits and disadvantages – and be in a better position to respond.

Outline of the chapters

The book is divided into two parts, focusing on theoretical perspectives and policies on consumerism, and on the manifestations of consumerism, and the experiences of 'consumers', respectively. Any division of an edited collection is bound to be somewhat arbitrary. As you will discover, some of the material covered in the chapters in Part I could just as easily have been placed in Part II, and vice versa. However, the chapters can be broadly divided in this way. Our aim has been to include contributions that offer critical and theoretical insights into the phenomenon of consumerism and its policy contexts, and contemporary empirical examples of how consumerism manifests in practice in various arenas of health care and is experienced by users of health care. While the perspectives offered in the individual chapters are diverse, the broad approach is sociological.

In Chapter 1, Arthur Frank sets the scene for the chapters that follow by asking: 'What's wrong with medical consumerism?' By juxtaposing two images of medicine – that of the empathic doctor, epitomized in Sir Luke Fildes's nineteenth-century painting, 'The Doctor', and a recent magazine advertisement for plastic and reconstructive surgery – Frank underlines the nature and impact of consumerism in medicine. As he indicates, the influence of medical consumerism has been profound and widespread. He outlines how medical consumerism has fashioned our understandings of health and the body, and self and society, and how it is used 'to reinforce the neo-liberalism of the high-intensity market'. As Frank concludes, despite the pervasiveness of medical consumerism, resistance is not futile. Sociologists can contribute to countering fatalism surrounding medical consumerism by offering an antidote: analysing its discourse.

In Chapter 2, Rob Irvine contributes to such an analysis by tracing the emergence of the 'health consumer' as a political concept. As Irvine argues, the category of 'health consumer' has been mobilized for both resistance and opposition to professional and bureaucratic power and provides a basis for policy development and the reinforcement of professional dominance. As this chapter clearly indicates, the concept 'health consumer' may be appropriated at different times for particular purposes. For example, in Australia, from the 1970s onwards, the consumer metaphor assisted patient advocacy and user groups in their efforts to gain greater social equality, but more recently it has served managerial reform in health care and the penetration of the state into the professional domain. As Irvine concludes, the arguments of consumer advocates should not be assumed to represent a radical break from the past.

The strategic deployment of the language of consumerism is clearly evident in the development of health consumer groups (otherwise known as patients' groups) in the UK – the focus of Chapter 3. In this chapter, Judith Allsop, Rob Baggott and Kathryn Jones examine a number of sociological and political theories that are pertinent to analysing the role of these groups in the national policy process. They draw on the findings of the first stage of a study which investigates how the groups involve their members in decision-making and participate in the policy-making process with politicians, professionals and business interests. Some of the claims about the role of such groups in the process of democratization and the development of 'social capital' can be challenged. While such groups have a strong ethos of involvement, and are routinely involved in bodies which formulate and implement health policy, different groups are not involved equally in decision-making, and the ability of consumer groups in general to affect policy agendas is questionable.

In Chapter 4, Pekka Sulkunen examines the shift in society from an emphasis on 'pastoral' power (i.e. care for the health and welfare of citizens) to consumer sovereignty (management of the self). Taking alcohol control in the Nordic countries as a case study and 'the flagship of the state's concern for citizens' health and welfare', Sulkunen traces the move from rigorous state control over alcohol, reflecting 'pastoral' regimes of power, to the consumer society of neo-liberalism. He identifies three waves of alcohol policy liberalism, each of which has changed the relationships between private life and the state and reflected different notions of freedom. The ethos of consumer society, argues Sulkunen, extends the managerial logic of the market to all aspects of life. In conclusion, he raises the question of whether the shifts in governmental rationality described for alcohol control are evident in other branches of the welfare state.

The final chapter in Part I – Chapter 5 by Mike Hazelton and Michael Clinton – draws attention to the limits of consumer participation in policy development in the area of mental health, which they attribute to problems inherent in the consumerism model itself. They describe a workshop project aiming to involve consumers in setting the future directions for the education and training of the mental health professions in Australia, and offer some reasons for the shortcomings of participation in practice. These include bureaucratic and professional dominance, a historically entrenched ethos in health care institutions of management and protection of the mentally ill, and the emergence of a 'post-liberal' order involving new forms of surveillance and exclusion. Finally, they question how mental health personnel might be managing the new policy directions.

In Part II, the reader is given a guided tour of a myriad of manifestations of consumerism and the experiences of 'consumers', ranging from the hospital setting and health care clinics to the general community. Chapter 6 by Saras Henderson addresses the experiences of patients in hospital. The chapter focuses on how aspects of the hospital context – including economic constraints, the culture of medical dominance and the prevalence of technology – work against the realization of consumerism in care. It draws upon the findings of an Australian study of patients' and nurses' perspectives on care in hospitals. The chapter challenges the rhetoric of the ideal of consumerism and argues that health care professionals have a long way to go before consumerism can be a reality in the practice setting.

Chapter 7, by Alan Petersen, Renata Kokanovic and Susan Hansen, describes how consumerism impacts on the carers of the mentally ill in a culturally diverse society. The chapter begins by outlining recent changes in the field of mental health care and the limits of the consumerism model in practice – a point that was also emphasized by Mike Hazelton and Michael Clinton in Chapter 5. Drawing on a recent Australian study of carers of the mentally ill in culturally and linguistically diverse communities, it provides a critical perspective on the manner in which carers of the mentally ill negotiate their way through the health care system. The chapter concludes with a recommendation to challenge the language of consumerism in mental health care policy.

In Chapter 8, Margaret Reid and Alexander Clark provide us with an interesting perspective on how consumer culture plays its part in the management of chronic illness, focusing on heart failure. Much of the literature focuses on issues of 'non-compliance', which suggests the notion of the passive patient, thus denying the active agency that is inherent in 'self-care'. Using empirical data from Scotland, Reid and Clark provide insight into the hard work involved in such management, in medication-taking and self-monitoring, which, contrary to the rhetoric of consumerism, is often a shared endeavour rather than an individual endeavour. As they explain, the concept of shared work has been little explored in the literature on chronic illness, yet for many sufferers the effort to achieve normality is a joint task, discussed and implemented by the sufferer and their partners.

Chapter 9, by Anthony Pryce, opens the door to a busy sexual health men's clinic in central London. Drawing on data derived from a study of two sexual health clinics, he provides us with an ethnographic account of sexual stories and consumer desires in which the discourse of sexualities and medicine is played out. The chapter describes the processes of consumption of sexual health services by clients who frequent the clinic, in particular the strategies employed by users in negotiating their encounters with clinic staff. Again, the theme of the active patient is deployed, with the chapter showing how the language of consumerism in the clinic reflects values and practices evident in the broader culture and informs clients' uptake and use of services.

In Chapter 10, Elizabeth Ettorre and Steven Miles focus attention on young people, drug use and the consumption of health. The authors challenge the normal discourse of youth and consumption, claiming that society's tendency to focus on young people as risk-takers or as risky consumers is problematic. The chapter illustrates the limitations of a pathological model of youth to young people's health consumption in relation to drug services, which fails to take account of the pleasurable aspects of young people's patterns of consumption. The authors emphasize the need to view young people's consumption of both drugs and drug services in light of the specific social locations that they occupy. In other words, there is a need to develop a 'youth-sensitive' approach to young people as consumers of drug services.

Finally, Chapter 11, by Robin Bunton and Paul Crawshaw, takes us to the commercial market of men's health consumption via the men's magazine *FHM* (*For Him Magazine*). This chapter shows how the culture of consumerism is perpetuated through such popular media forms. Employing the method of discourse analysis, the authors examine competing and often contradictory discourses of the male body and men's health. Comparison is also made between men's and women's magazines in relation to health and health consumption. Men's magazines reflect the existence of multiple masculine identities, and present readers with contradictory cultural values relating to good citizenship and masculinity.

References

Barry, A., Osborne, T. and Rose, N. (1996) *Foucault and Political Reason: Liberalism, Neo-Liberalism and Rationalities of Government*, London: UCL Press Ltd.

Baudrillard, J. (1998) *The Consumer Society: Myths and Structures*, London: Sage.

Bauman, Z. (1998) *Work, Consumerism and the New Poor*, Buckingham and Philadelphia: Open University Press.

Brock, S.C. (1995) 'Narrative and medical genetics: on ethics and therapeutics', *Qualitative Health Research*, 5: 150–68.

Bunton, R. and Burrows, R. (1995) 'Consumption and health in the "epidemiological" clinic of late modern medicine', in R. Bunton, S. Nettleton and R. Burrows (eds) *The Sociology of Health Promotion: Critical Analyses of Consumption, Lifestyle and Risk*, London and New York: Routledge.

Burchell, G., Gordon, C. and Miller, P. (1991) *The Foucault Effect: Studies in Governmentality*, Hemel Hempstead: Harvester Wheatsheaf.

Corrigan, P. (1997) *The Sociology of Consumption*, London: Sage.

Falk, P. (1994) *The Consuming Body*, London: Sage.

Featherstone, M. (1991) 'The body in consumer culture', in M. Featherstone, M. Hepworth and B.S. Turner (eds) *The Body: Social Process and Cultural Theory*, London: Sage.

Frank, A.W. (2000) 'All the things which do not fit: Baudrillard and medical consumerism', *Families, Systems and Health*, 18, 2: 205–16.

Grace, V.M. (1991) 'The marketing of empowerment and the construction of the health consumer: a critique of health promotion', *International Journal of Health Services*, 21, 2: 329–43.

—— (1994) 'What is a health consumer?', in C. Waddell and A.R. Petersen (eds) *Just Health: Inequality in Illness, Care and Prevention*, Melbourne: Churchill Livingstone.

Hogg, C. (1999) *Patients, Power and Politics: From Patients to Citizens*, London: Sage.

Hugman, R. (1994) 'Consuming health and welfare', in R. Keat, N. Whitely and N. Abercrombie (eds) *The Authority of the Consumer*, London and New York: Routledge.

Keat, R., Whitely, N. and Abercrombie, N. (eds) (1994) *The Authority of the Consumer*, London and New York: Routledge.

Lee, M.J. (ed.) (2000) *The Consumer Society Reader*, Massachusetts, Malden: Blackwell Publishers Ltd.

Lupton, D. (1997) 'Consumerism, reflexivity and the medical encounter', *Social Science and Medicine*, 45, 3: 373–81.

Lupton, D., Donaldson, C. and Lloyd, P. (1991) 'Caveat emptor or blissful ignorance? Patients and the consumerist ethos', *Social Science and Medicine*, 33, 5: 559–68.

Miles, S. (1998) *Consumerism – as a Way of Life*, London: Sage.

Miller, D. (2001) *Consumption*, London: Routledge.

Rose, N. (1999) *Powers of Freedom: Reframing Political Thought*, Cambridge: Cambridge University Press.

Shackely, P. and Ryan, M. (1994) 'What is the role of the consumer in health care?', *Journal of Social Policy*, 23, 4: 517–41.

Spivak, G.C. (1993) *Outside the Teaching Machine*, New York: Routledge.

Sulkunen, P., Holmwood, J., Radner, H. and Schulze, G. (eds) (1997) *Constructing the New Consumer Society*, Houndmills, Basingstoke: Macmillan Press Ltd.

Urry, J. (1995) *Consuming Places*, London and New York: Routledge.

Part I

Consumerism in context

Theoretical perspectives and policies

Chapter 1

What's wrong with medical consumerism?

Arthur W. Frank

The juxtaposition of two images of medicine begins to suggest what has changed. The first is a late nineteenth-century painting (later an engraving) by Sir Luke Fildes, entitled 'The Doctor'. Physician Alfred Tauber, who chose it as the cover for his recent meditation on medicine and its ethics, describes the painting and its significance as an icon of medicine:

> This Victorian pastoral drama shows a country doctor sitting contemplatively [leaning forward at a 45 degree angle, one hand supporting his chin; the figure is utterly still yet poised to move forward] at the bedside of a sick child, whose parents look on in dismay and fear. Portraying the medical reality of that period just before the explosion of scientific medicine, Fildes's evocation of the empathic doctor, helpless in the face of nature's ravage and yet steadfastly committed to remaining with his young patient, both reflected the sentimentality of that era and also stated clearly the ethical relationship of the physician to his charge ... Today, the painting still occupies a prominent place at the Tate Gallery in London, and I think it commands attention not so much for its large size and effective naturalism but more so because Fildes captured a human relation that is of time immemorial, and we respond instinctively to his depiction of this relation. The painting is a powerful image of my own philosophy of medicine – not the posture of a helpless physician watching the relentless scourge of nature, but the physician as empathic witness.
>
> (Tauber 1999: 106–7)

I once saw Fildes's painting presented as a slide at a medical meeting, and the audience response leads me to generalize Tauber's interpretation. To physicians dealing with the restraints of managed care on the one hand, and the expanding frontiers of medical services on the other, the painting offers nostalgia for a medicine in which technical practices may have been primitive by contemporary standards but goals and ethics can seem uncomplicated in their idealism.

Disease in Tauber's gloss of the painting is 'nature's ravage' and 'the relentless scourge of nature'. The patient is most emphatically not a 'consumer' in any sense of that world; her life is in danger. The physician opposes nature with few resources at his (the appropriate pronoun for the time) disposal, but what he lacks in interventive technology he makes up in 'empathic witness'. Tauber realizes that many contemporary physicians would regard the painting as 'the posture of a helpless physician', and he deflects this interpretation. For him the primacy of the caring relationship occasioned by human vulnerability to nature is the enduring significance of the painting. Medicine is founded on the recognition of human suffering: when the physician can no longer cure, he continues to care.

The history of Tauber's own relationship to the painting does not exactly undercut his interpretation but suggests the fragility of his version of the image. His father, also a physician, was given a reproduction of 'The Doctor' by 'a pharmaceutical house'. 'Knowing my attachment to this lithograph hanging in his waiting room,' Tauber writes, 'he gave me a small three-dimensional porcelain facsimile of the scene – also supplied by the drug company' (1999: 106). The caring relationship of father to son mirrors that of physician to patient, yet a third party has intervened: the drug company that produced both reproductions and distributed them as gifts to physicians. New pharmaceuticals would render the fever watch of Fildes's physician (happily) obsolete, but writing a prescription would increasingly (and perhaps less happily) replace the 'empathic witness' that Tauber idealizes. In distributing the image as a publicity give-away, the drug company commodified nostalgia for a kind of medical practice that it itself was instrumental in ending, for better and for worse.

I move forward more than a century to a very different image: an advertisement on the inside back cover of a new Australian-American magazine, *The Art of Cosmetic Beauty*, which had its inaugural issue in Summer 2000. The magazine is 8.5 inches by 11.5 inches, printed on high-quality paper providing excellent resolution to its graphics; its price and production values elevate it above supermarket check-out 'beauty' magazines.

The advertisement is for the services of Dr R, Plastic and Reconstructive Surgery.[1] The centre of the image, 7.5 inches, is a portrait of Dr R. He looks straight at the camera with a slight smile, hands on hips, wearing bright blue surgical scrubs (looking fresh from the laundry) with a surgical cap and mask (open, worn around his neck). On the upper border (just under 2 inches) is the copy: 'When the eye of a gifted artist and the hand of a skilled surgeon come together, every part of you can be more beautiful.' Down the side borders (with Dr R's elbows blocking parts of some images) are six photographs of parts of women's bodies: eye, hip, abdomen, shoulder and breast (discretely in shadow), full face, and nose and mouth. The bottom border specifies his name, Board Certification, services ('Facial Rejuvenation, Breast Augmentation, Liposuction, Endermologie$^{(TM)}$'), address, and – a ubiquitous feature of such advertising – his website. The bottom line of the image says, all in capitals: 'Call to schedule your complimentary consultation.'

The last line is particularly interesting since, in another article, readers are warned by Dr Harlan Pollock, identified as 'chair of the Public Education Committee of the American Society of Plastic Surgeons', that 'Free consultations are a gimmick that are used in obtaining patients and they're worth about what they cost ... . They are an opportunity to sell an operation and serve very little purpose' (Bishop 2000a: 87). The apparent contradiction between this caveat in the text of an article and the advertising image is typical of magazines generally and of *The Art of Cosmetic Beauty* particularly. The editorial introduction to the first issue specifies, 'Never far from our articles will be the message that surgery is surgery and any reputable surgeon will tell you that procedures can enhance the way one looks but it [sic] doesn't alter the person' (Grujovic 2000: 6). That message is repeated throughout even as it is undercut by advertising copy such as that on the back cover: 'Celebrate a reflection of the true you by scheduling a consultation with Dr W ... medical professionals dedicated to helping you discover your beautiful side.'

In the transition from Fildes's doctor to the cosmetic surgeon, the image of medicine shifts from Tauber's empathic witness to the 'gifted artist' with the surgical skills to shape the human body to his aesthetic vision. 'Nature', as the object of the physician's work, ceases to be what Tauber calls 'ravage and scourge' and becomes instead the raw material awaiting the human intervention that will perfect it.

Fildes's physician gazes at his sleeping patient, alert to whatever he can do – probably nothing – that might affect the outcome. Dr R, the cosmetic surgeon, is surrounded by fragments of beautiful women. In the synecdoche of these images, the perfection of each fragment creates the imagination of a plenitude that includes not only perfect bodies but perfect 'lifestyles'. There need be no direct statement specifying that the photos of women surrounding Dr R are the outcome of his work; this association is less than crucial. The message is that the body's wholeness and happiness lies in the perfection of each of its parts. In beauty the 'true you' is simultaneously released and invented. Thus the surgeon no longer contemplates human suffering; rather he perfects contingent imperfection. Fildes's physician seems to wonder what he can possibly do; Dr R stands ready to show his next patient how much he can do.

What is to be made of this juxtaposition of images? Critique risks lapsing into a moralism (whether neo-Marxist or neo-Calvinist) that can become what psychiatrist Peter Kramer (2000) calls 'the valorization of sadness'. Kramer, it should be noted, is author of the best-selling *Listening to Prozac* in which he coined the term 'cosmetic psychopharmacology'. He builds a compelling case that there is a long-standing critical bias that identifies the serious (in whatever cultural field) with the sad. Happiness, in itself, is often regarded as trivial.

The critique of medical consumerism is not about the triviality or authenticity of the individual lives of people who seek and purchase these services. The object of critique is the society in which these services are offered as they are. Sociological interpretation begins from the counterintuitive presupposition that the effects of medical consumerism may ultimately be as great, and possibly greater, on those who do *not* themselves receive these services but who live in a society of which these services are a part. What counts is how common-sense perception of bodies and lives are affected by the publicizing of available services.

Most discussions of medical consumerism take a should-they-or-shouldn't-they perspective. Individual decisions to seek or not to seek commodities were understood by Georg Simmel (in his 1903 essay, 'The Metropolis and Mental Life') as part of a historical tendency by which 'individuals who had been liberated from their historical bonds sought now to distinguish themselves from one another' (1971: 339). 'Regardless of whether we are sympathetic or antipathetic with their individual expressions,' Simmel concluded, 'they transcend the sphere in which a judge-like attitude on our part is appropriate.' What counted for Simmel was to study 'the totality of historical life to which we belong'. The point is neither 'to complain or to condone' individual acts but 'to understand' their place in that totality (1971: 339). Thus my concern is not with the true motives of individual consumers, but rather with consumption as an increasingly prevalent social discourse that legitimates a variety of attitudes and practices (Wernick 1991).

Simmel's rejection of complaining or condoning does not, as I read him, imply abandoning critique. How society complains about and condones medical consumerism seems crucial in the future of the historical totality that I will follow others in calling neo-liberalism. If the most salient characteristic of neo-liberal society is its capacity to assert itself as not having any viable alternative (Bourdieu 1998), then developing a critique of medical consumerism is a crucial demonstration of the continuing possibility of critique itself.

In asking what's wrong with medical consumerism I present attempts to purchase cosmetic beauty as my primary examples with the recognition that these practices may become an increasingly minor part of the medical consumerist future. Genetic interventions seem poised to be the dominant form of consumerism and are the issue of concern among leading bioethicists (Buchanan *et al.* 2000) as well as disability activists (reviewed by Parens and Asch 1999). If the promissory notes of the new genetics have any validity, we can imagine a clinic advertisement in the next decade or two that might read: 'When the dreams of parents and the right genetic technology come together, your child can enjoy every opportunity life offers.' The question of this future has high stakes for medicine and for society. Economic interests and technical possibility will create this future, but perhaps critiques can act – in Weber's famous metaphor of 1913 – as switchmen, deflecting the course of this future slightly but consequentially (Weber 1958: 280).

Beauty as medical commodity

We would hardly expect to find the word 'consumerism' in *The Art of Cosmetic Beauty*, but what is surprising is how completely the whole aspect of payment for products and services is rendered invisible. Even articles specifically devoted to the promotion of 'products' ('face, body, hair, make-up' and later, dental) do not mention prices. One of the few places where dollar signs can be found is in a fascinating set of 'recommendations' for the age (by decade) when different 'skin changes' occur and what interventions are recommended; thus: '30s Blotchiness, frown lines, crow's feet, forehead wrinkles. Treatment: Use Botox, approx. $500' (Muzik 2000: 66; prices presumably in US dollars). An article comparing the benefits of 'Blue Peel treatment' to laser resurfacing ($200–$800 versus $2,500–$5,000; Bishop 2000b: 70) and a couple of mentions of spa treatments are, on my perusal, the only other places where it is suggested that payments are made. Thus, at the high end of consumerism, what for Simmel was the underlying form of the activity – the money economy – is set discretely out of view.[2]

In medicine as elsewhere, first-world consumerism is often most explicit when viewed in the mirror of third-world adaptations; thus to locate the act of consuming I turn to a recent report of cosmetic surgery in Iran. 'So a cool thing to do in Tehran these days is to get a nose job,' reports *The New York Times*.

> So cool that unlike women in many places, who hide the chiseling and sawing and stretching done to their faces, Iranian women wear their post-surgical bandages like badges of honor, or at least indicators of a certain wealth.
>
> (Sciolino 2000)

The description points towards an operational definition of the dense keyword, *consumerism*. As the post-surgical bandages themselves become worth wearing, the surgical enterprise takes a reflexive twist. The surgery is not only the instrumental means to achieve a desired end; surgery itself is also a desired end, as a display of wealth.

The Iranian report also offers some remarkably candid statements of what is desired from surgery. In these we hear the voices of consumers, however ungeneralizable. I quote these women not to suggest that what they say reveals the truth of their motivations, but rather for these quotations' expression of the discourse of consumerism. The quotation of these voices in *The New York Times* will doubtless be read differently by different readers: some will regard the *Times* engaged in a neo-colonialist deprecation of the Third World, other readers will find legitimation of their own attitude towards medical consumerism, and still others will read the quotations as I do, actually saying what Westerns act upon but are reticent to express.

> The mother of a 17-year-old whose nose had been changed surgically said: 'We did her nose so she could become more beautiful and enjoy her face for the rest of her life. I could see that she had a flaw in her face, and I was very glad we could get rid of it.'

> 'Unfortunately, in my family everyone has bad noses', said a 20-year-old called Haleh after she had had her nose shrunk. 'This is a very, very serious flaw. Their faces change after the operation. They suddenly look beautiful. So all our family members are very sensitive about the shape of our noses, and everywhere we go we make comments about people's noses.'

> 'I want a smaller nose, like a doll's nose', [Ms Moghimi] said. 'I'm willing to pay lots of money to a plastic surgeon to give me a new look. I don't want to have any faults in my face. I'd like to look beautiful, like Marilyn Monroe.'
>
> (Sciolino 2000)

These statements provide at least three parameters to consumerism in general. First is the pleasure of spending money. As these women are quoted, they seem somewhere between the ideal type that Simmer called the spendthrift, for whom 'the pleasure of waste depends simply on the expenditure of money for no-matter-what objects' (1971: 182) and Veblen's ([1899] 1953) understanding of conspicuous consumption as acts of displaying wealth. There is pleasure in wearing the bandages as well as pleasure in the reconstructed face.

Second we can hear intimations of what Simmel called 'the curse of restlessness and transience ... every pleasure attained arouses the desire for further pleasure, which can never be satisfied' (1971: 185). Reading what the Iranian women say, I am not alone in wondering how long it will be before other 'flaws' have to be got 'rid of'. That the whole body awaits improvement – and, with age, constant improvement – is evident on one surgeon's website (described by *The Art of Cosmetic Beauty* as 'very reader friendly – fun and informative' (McCloskey 2000: 34)) where the homepage features an idealized nude woman (simulated or real? a cartoon or the result of surgery? who can tell, and who bothers to ask?) with the invitation to click on part of her body to learn about surgery to that area. The *Times* quotes an Iranian cosmetic surgeon (American trained) saying: 'What's in fashion right now is getting the nose done. After that come face-lifts' (Sciolino 2000).

The third parameter I want to single out – among others that could be observed – is that consumerism individualizes the bases and morality of action. The self is the sole referent. In particular the consumer defines money as his or her exclusive resource to expend as she or he chooses. In the following quotation, also from Ms Moghimi, quoted above, a narrative account that initially points in the direction of culture turns to focus on the isolated self:

> 'Part of the reason for spending so much attention on the way I look is that it's in our culture. ... It's in the nature of Iranian women to want to look beautiful. Part of the reason is that I don't have anything else to do. My only job is to cook and take care of my home. So I spend time [and money, as stated in the earlier quotation of Ms Moghimi] on myself'.
>
> (Sciolino 2000)

Neo-liberalism elevates consumer choice to the level of a right that society is organized to defend; the right of each to spend his or her own resources as he or she chooses is the organizing principle behind the privatization of government services. 'Giving money back' to taxpayer/consumers and allowing them to spend it *as they choose* is the recurring slogan of neo-liberal political parties. Advertisements by cosmetic surgeons join this presumption of consumer right with psychotherapeutic imperatives to discover or liberate an inner self that has been repressed or hidden; thus messages such as the one quoted above, 'celebrate a reflection of the true you'. That the celebration has to be paid for does not go entirely without saying, since many websites include an 'online financing' link.

Many Western consumers of cosmetic beauty would doubtless find the quotations of the Iranian women embarrassing. For them the Fall/Winter 2000 catalogue of The Body Shop, an international merchandiser of beauty products, offers the message of celebration a spiritual and eco-political twist: 'It's enlightenment, empowerment, activism. Knowing the score and wanting more. We're talking all-round well-being – in body and soul, in our communities and in our global environment.' Body Shop products 'incorporate the wisdom of world communities and the knowledge of the ages'. The Canadian version of this catalogue ends its introductory message with a note about hours of 'paid staff time' donated to violence-prevention programmes and the amount of money raised for these programmes.

The Body Shop's publicity exemplifies and legitimates two central tenets of neo-liberal ideology. First, any meaningful social action can only occur through volunteer activity with corporate sponsorship; 'partnership' is the current buzzword. The idea of government is conspicuously absent; it is *not* worth stating how much The Body Shop paid in corporate taxes that sustain government services. What Zygmunt Bauman calls 'Politics with a capital P' (2000: 70) has dropped out of the discourse of social improvement; in its place, buying at The Body Shop is depicted as the means to the good society. Thus the second neo-liberal tenet: social progress occurs through globalized trade. The catalogue features 'the power of community economic initiatives to effect positive change' in their 'Community Trade programme'. Shoppers are invited to 'discover some of the world's most amazing natural ingredients grown through traditional practices'. Bauman expresses the most sceptical interpretation of this message and the practices of production and consumption behind it: 'The freedom to treat the whole of life as one protracted shopping spree means casting the world as a warehouse overflowing with consumer commodities' (2000: 89). In The Body Shop catalogue, this warehouse includes 'the knowledge of the ages' as well as 'amazing natural ingredients' the purity of which is guaranteed by 'traditional practices'.

What most critics would attack in either *The Art of Cosmetic Beauty* or The Body Shop catalogue is the merging of needs and wants. Medical consumerism renders the needs/wants distinction ambiguous because the same medical service often addresses both wants that seem utterly discretionary and needs that seem as real as that of the patient in Fildes's painting. *The Art of Cosmetic Beauty* includes an article on corrective surgery with a subtitle reading: 'Cosmetic surgery is not only a matter of vanity. For some it is a necessity. Approximately 12,000 children are born in the US each year suffering from a cleft palate or deformity of the head and face' (Bishop and Stapleton 2000: 98). As before-and-after photos of surgeries transforming badly deformed babies' faces into 'normal' happy children mix with those removing wrinkles, presumably some of the wrinkled would argue that their condition too is not vanity but necessity.[3]

The ambiguity over which are 'necessary' cases leads to the more extensive question, crucial to the critique of consumerism, of whether any experienced need can be judged false or manipulated.

The social mediation of need

'Consumerism' takes its pejorative force from an underlying assumption that people either seek to fulfil real needs with unsatisfactory objects, or they are manipulated by producers into pursuing false needs. In an argument that remains current despite being twenty-five years old, William Leiss (1976: 53) suggests three 'patterns of thinking about needs'.

The first pattern includes arguments that attempt to distinguish biological from cultural needs; the objective is often to establish some category of 'basic human needs'. Leiss argues, convincingly on my reading, that like all attempts to separate nature from culture, this effort fails. Citing anthropologist Dorothy Lee, Leiss (1976: 54) argues that

> needs themselves are derivative, not basic. They are not the underlying foundations which explain the orientation of individual behaviour, but rather are themselves derived from a more fundamental set of values, varying [perhaps less in the age of the Internet] from culture to culture.[4]

The second pattern includes attempts to establish a hierarchy of needs 'said to have differing degrees of urgency and significance' (1976: 55). Leiss shows that establishing such hierarchies requires, like the argument above, positing dichotomies of nature/biology versus culture. These dichotomies ignore the contextualizing force of what he calls the 'high-intensity market' (1976: 57). In societies based on such markets, 'The needs of self-esteem and self-actualization are expressed and pursued through the purchase of commodities, which are not simply material objects but things that have a complex set of meanings of "messages" associated with them' (1976: 57). The conventional claim is that market forces intervene via some form of advertising to distort people's sense of what is self-actualizing. Leiss suggests that in high-intensity-market societies the ideal of self-actualization is always already 'expressed and pursued' through commodities.

The final pattern argues that needs are distorted by social processes, e.g. socialization and the market economy. While Leiss readily acknowledges that the market endlessly seeks to manipulate needs, he points out that this manipulation does not in itself render those needs false. He returns to a variant of his earlier argument: 'All wants arise out of social conditioning ... individuals learn to interpret their needs and to adjust themselves to prevailing modes of approved behaviour' (1976: 58).

Though he does treat the high-intensity market as a contextual condition not likely to change, Leiss's argument is not neo-liberalism *avant la lettre*. He is clear that 'individuals become increasingly confused about the relationship between their needs and the means through which they try to satisfy them' (1976: 63). What he is arguing against is the possibility of doing what many bioethicists currently hope to accomplish: 'develop fixed and abstract categories' that would distinguish real needs from false ones (1976: 60). The problem for Leiss is not false needs but a market environment that makes it increasingly difficult for individuals who necessarily lack sufficient information about most if not all the products and services they purchase to interpret 'the relationship between their perceived needs and the possible sources of satisfaction for them' (1976: 63).

Leiss (1976: 93) forces critics of consumerism to acknowledge that needs and objects define each other, reciprocally and recursively. While some needs certainly have greater intensity than others at certain moments – Fildes's 'The Doctor' depicts such a moment – attempts to fix categories of real, objective needs versus false, manipulated needs fail to acknowledge that social schemes of value precede any such distinctions.[5] To ask whether bodies in the 'before' photos of cosmetic surgeons *needed* fixing – to seek categories that fix the 'flaws' that are worthy of fixing – engages in what Leiss calls 'Sunday sermons' (1976: 57) designed to assert one aesthetic – one preferred form of life – over another.

Of course any person intuitively feels that some needs are real and others are false. Thus I immediately perceive surgery correcting babies' facial deformities as meeting a real need and I am cynical about what *The New York Times* writer Elaine Sciolino (2000) calls 'chiseling and sawing and stretching' to improve what is already (as I see it) a 'normal' appearance. Leiss's anthropology-based argument requires recognizing that my common-sense response, like any understanding of human needs, will always be socially mediated. This inevitability of social mediation does not mean, however, that any particular form of mediation is above critique; depending on one's ethical criteria, some forms of mediation can be judged preferable to others. Thus the question of what's wrong with medical consumerism becomes two intertwined questions. First, how is reshaping the understanding of 'health' crucial to the specific mediation of needs that is typical of neo-liberal societies at this historical moment in those societies? Second, what negative effects does this neo-liberal mediation of needs have?

Distorting bodies, medicine and society

Three critiques of medical consumerism are hardly exhaustive but seem fundamental. The first level of critique concerns the body. The conventional criticism is that body consumerism is manipulated by messages that pair images of an ideal body with a product that promises to close the gap between the consumer's body and that ideal. Critics argue that the ideal is an aberration (for example, the super-model) and probably also a fabrication as well (the photos have been retouched); thus body images and needs are being manipulated. A response interpolated from Leiss is that such criticism – while descriptively accurate of marketing practices – ignores that any culture has its dominant aesthetic of bodies and so any body image always already confronts a gap between itself and some ideal. A response could be that contemporary advertising strategically manipulates that gap. Still, the accusing critics *depend no less* than the accused manipulators on presupposing some *a priori* body: the natural, unmanipulated body presupposed by the critics is no less idealized than the commodity-enhanced body of the manipulators. As I observe incitements to medical consumerism, their capacity for distortion lies less in presenting a false ideal (though it may be false) but in obliterating *any* coherent sense of the body image. Incitements may begin with some idealized image but this image soon deconstructs, leaving only endless fragmentation.

The ideal bodies of models (in photos that seem to call attention to being computer enhanced) do invite consumers to websites. But cosmetic surgery websites show few ideal bodies; because the pin-up image of the woman's body that serves as a link to different surgical services (by clicking on part of her) is such an exception that most viewers will probably see it as a joke. The vast majority of website images are detailed fragments of bodies – the before-and-after shots of body parts.[6] The extreme clinical detail of these images gives bodies a new literalness, not a fantasy perfection.

One effect of the accumulated fragmentation is to efface any referent – natural or ideal – of a whole body. Fragmentation renders the body perpetually unstable; no body can ever be idealized because the fragments never compose into a coherent whole. Of course the body's 'coherence' is always an idealization – and as critics of advertising point out, a dangerous one in some respects. However unreachable the telos of the body's coherence, it provides one basis of the telos of the self's coherence – equally unreachable but nonetheless important as an ideal. The body-in-fragments reduces the telos of coherence to perpetual shopping for marginally improved parts.

Some form of commodification of the body is to be expected in what Leiss calls a high-intensity-market society. The problem is not that the body is commodified; rather the problem is a form of commodification that requires fragmentation in order to assign a cash value to each increment of improvement of each part. Leiss's description of the effect of fragmentation remains the best articulation of how cosmetic surgical websites do not distort bodies themselves but do distort lives:

> Thus the expression of need itself is progressively fragmented into smaller and smaller bits ... . The constant redivision and recombination of need-fragments renders it increasingly difficult, if not impossible, for individuals to develop a coherent set of objectives for their needs and thus to make judgments about the suitability of particular goods for them.
>
> (Leiss 1976: 88)

What is distorted is the possibility of living a coherent life *as* the body that a person is.

Leiss's critique of fragmentation anticipates Richard Sennett's (1998) evaluation of the 'corrosion of character' in contemporary conditions of work life. For Sennett corrosion results from the absence of the possibilities for temporally coherent careers and what he calls 'legible' work functions. Unsure of what they will be doing tomorrow, or exactly what their work today actually accomplishes, people cannot develop a coherent set of objectives for their lives or make judgements about the suitability of their next career and family choices. Their sense of what they value about themselves, and how they are valuable to each other, corrodes. Their lives lack a coherent narrative (Sennett 1998: 24ff).

Medical consumerism does not so much distort people's images of their bodies; as I suggest above, it may provide many people with far more literal images of many more real bodies. However, the fragmentation of the body into images, necessary for commodifying the body, can distort people's character because character is embodied. In the constant instability of these fragments – i.e. never coming together as a whole – character is corroded because people lose the coherence that begins in the body and is sustained (if always partially unrealized) in the body. When Alfred Schutz observed that 'we grow old together' (1971: 220), he recognized that a person's experiences of his or her own body ageing, set amid mutual perceptions of other's bodies ageing, are a fundamental condition of intersubjectivity. The capacities for setting coherent objectives and making judgement about acts in a world of others – the capacity for character in Sennett's terms – depend on believing in the coherence of one's own body amid other bodies.

To summarize my first level of critique, fragmentation distorts because it renders bodies like other merchandised commodities: collections of 'features'. Homes, cars and stereos are now advertised with a bulleted list of their features; the number of features sets one version of a commodity above another. As transformed by the language of merchandising, 'homes' are no longer places that achieve value through the accumulated experiences of lives transpiring there but instead become collections of features – hot tubs, bars, decks, views, and so forth. Features can be added and upgraded, enhancing value. Cosmetic surgery fragments the body into a set of features that can be serially upgraded. The full importance of imposing the language of merchandising on the body is not that cash value is inherently degrading; Leiss seems right in granting the capacity of the high-intensity market to put a price tag on anything. The point is that if genetic engineering is anything more than a fantasy, the decomposition of the body into features is preparing for that future. Far more consequential than upgrading the ageing features of the adult body may be preselecting features in the embryonic body and changing DNA structure in order to do this.

My second critique of medical consumerism is that it distorts perceptions of medicine as a social good. Again, Leiss's analysis of needs arguments renders the case for distortion less than self-evident by showing that it depends on contrasts between the all-too-evidently flawed present and a past idealized in such nostalgic objects as Fildes's 'The Doctor'. 'The Doctor' gives self-evidence to the idea that medicine once had, and could again have, a core mission that is pure and unquestionable. Tauber's gloss on Fildes's painting, quoted above, can now be reread as depending on its explicit opposition between the nature that brings the ravages of disease and the physician who, as a representative of culture, opposes nature. The physician opposes the ravages of nature (bad, unnatural nature) and seeks to restore his patient to her natural health (good nature).

The idea that medicine ever had a pure mission that could be distorted in contemporary consumerism is rendered all the more questionable when we recall what some of the 1890s colleagues of Fildes's country physician were engaged in. Michel Foucault's (1976) history of sexuality recollects that the medicine of this period defined masturbation as a disease and engaged in horribly invasive surgery to 'cure' this ravage of nature. Medical historian Rachel Maines (1999) describes how the mechanical vibrator was developed during this same period as a medical device for use by physicians.[7] These examples are necessarily eclectic but can be found in any medical generation. The definition of health has never been based only on 'nature's ravages' as real as these are, but also on medicine's perceived capacities and market opportunities. Just as the body is always already socially mediated in its needs, so medicine has never had pure objectives transparently defined as responses to nature's unnatural moments.

The nostalgia aroused by Fildes's painting can also cause us to forget that physicians of that time collected fees for their services, at least from enough patients much of the time to compensate for those to whom care was offered *pro bono*. Perhaps the parents in Fildes's painting were charity cases, or perhaps somewhere in their worries was concern about how they were going to pay for this doctor's attention, however empathic it might be. A genuine social advance of the twentieth century was most countries' adoption of government health insurance guaranteeing some level of medical services to all regardless of ability to pay.

Medical consumerism may not threaten an abstract ideal of medicine, but at a time when, as Bauman (2000: 106) notes, 'the idea of "the common good" [has been] branded suspect, threatening, nebulous, or addle-brained', consumerism does erode the ideal that medicine can be one such common good. In neo-liberal' society an increasingly fragile public consensus supports the idea that medical goods are different from other goods traded in the market and the government has some responsibility to protect all citizens' access to these goods. Because a collective sense of responsibility for the vulnerable seems essential to sustaining the idea that society has common goods, here my argument shifts to a third level of critique, how medical consumerism distorts society.

The Art of Cosmetic Beauty is organized in sections which progress not only by degree of invasiveness but also by cost: 'Bottled Beauty' leads to 'the Non-Surgical section' (including laser skin treatments, for example). Then following the 'Dental' and 'Men's Only' (mostly on pectoral implants) sections comes, 'at the top of the ladder', the 'Surgical section' (Grujovic 2000: 6). The almost explicit message is that medical intervention is part of a continuum of products among which a consumer gets as much as he or she can afford. In the neo-liberal debates over provision of health care, this message quickly becomes generalized as the following example describes.

In January 2001 the Canadian Broadcasting Company news reported that another privately operated, fee-for-service magnetic resonance imaging (MRI) clinic opened in the Province of Quebec, intensifying a controversy between the provincial ministry of health and the federal Canadian government. The federal government maintains that all medical services that are publicly provided should *only* be publicly provided; the only private services will be those completely outside public provision (for example, most cosmetic surgery). 'Queue-jumping' goes against universalism. The neo-liberal counter-position was expressed by a Quebec physician who described the new clinic as giving patients 'another option'. That option is to pay for their own MRI scan, possibly receive early diagnosis, and move more quickly to treatment in the publicly-funded system. The federal government fears that provincial health ministries, whose budgets pay for public health care, will let waiting lists grow longer to push more people into private treatment. The neo-liberal response is that fee-for-service treatment shortens public waiting lists while allowing consumers to spend their money as they choose; those who can afford private treatment and those who cannot both receive better service.

Whether consumers progress from Bottled Beauty to Surgical interventions is genuinely optional in that none will live or die depending on whether they can exercise the option; one can choose to spend one's money elsewhere and possibly be healthier by doing so. Neo-liberalism then generalizes that perception of medical services as options to treatments like MRIs which can determine whether someone lives or dies.[8] Bourdieu's observation that neo-liberal ideology 'is based on a kind of social neo-Darwinism' (1998: 42) is literally true in health care. Of course no one would say that if the poor receive care later than the rich and die as a result, that's little loss; yet that brutal conclusion is inescapable.

Contemporary cosmetic interventions may, if anything, be detrimental to the health of their consumers.[9] These cosmetic interventions, however, create a milieu in which more medical goods, more of the time, are regarded as commodities which people have the option to purchase, just as they have options to purchase other commodities. Cosmetic interventions, and the publicity around them, also intensify the body as a site for more complex investments of capital. Here my argument returns to the Iranian women wearing their surgical bandages. Today's consumerism may end in conspicuous displays of the resources that the person can invest in the body – or some means of reconversion of this investment may be possible; for example, the Iranian daughter's now unflawed nose may display her as available for a more advantageous marriage that solidifies an economic alliance between families. But these displays of investment in beauty and the reconversion of those investments into other forms of capital can only provide what might be called secondary or derivative value; the perfected nose has no intrinsic value but only creates terms of recognition that can attract other values. The potential of genetic medicine is that investments might yield *direct* returns in enhancing the body's capacities and resistances. The most significant consumption value of genetic medicine will not be conspicuous but rather will provide significant competitive advantages precisely by being invisible.

Ultimately medical consumerism affects society by insinuating health as the contemporary basis of what Weber argued religion traditionally reinforced: 'the theodicy of good fortune'.

> In treating suffering as a symptom of odiousness in the eyes of the gods and as a sign of secret guilt, religion has psychologically met a very general need. The fortunate is seldom satisfied with the fact of being fortunate. Beyond this, he [sic] wants to be convinced that he has a *right* to his good fortune. He wants to be convinced that he 'deserves' it, and above all, that he deserves it in comparison with others.
>
> (Weber 1958: 271)

This general need that was once met by religion is now met by the political-economic orthodoxy of neo-liberalism, our contemporary theodicy of good fortune. Medical consumerism instantiates this good fortune in the body. This theodicy of good fortune requires believing that one has caused one's health and thus deserves it, just as others deserve whatever health they have caused. Davis (1995:163) emphasizes this sense of agency among the women she interviewed about having cosmetic surgery: 'In a context of limited possibilities for action, cosmetic surgery can be a way for an individual woman to give shape to her life by reshaping her body.' Given the ambivalent outcomes of their surgeries, the language of agency of these women could hardly be called a theodicy of *good* fortune, but it is a language in which one's fortune is what one brings about. As I have emphasized above, what counts is what this language prepares for. The literal embodiment of the theodicy of good fortune will be (not too distant) future parents speaking this same language of agency about their genetically perfected child, and that child believing that these purchased advantages are her or his birthright.

That future – contested as to its possibility as well as its desirability – is not yet here. Of the present state of medical consumerism, Davis may offer the most humane conclusion: 'For a woman whose suffering has gone beyond a certain point, cosmetic surgery can become a matter of justice – the only fair thing to do' (1995: 163; cf. 173). Perhaps behind the *The New York Times'* quotations of Iranian women there are untold stories of suffering. These stories are as serious as the stories of families with congenital diseases who anxiously await the possibility of genetic modifications (Beeson and Doksum 2001; Cox 1999). I began this essay by quoting Simmel. The objective is neither to complain about nor to condone individual choices; rather the objective is to understand how individuals shape the social totality that shapes their and others' choices, whether or not individuals intend to shape that totality.

Medical consumerism is being recreated, in ideology and substance, to reinforce the neo-liberalism of the high-intensity market. But resistance is not futile. Bourdieu (1998: 55) writes: 'We, as sociologists, without denouncing anyone, can undertake to map out these networks and show how the circulation of ideas is subtended by a circulation of power.' Bourdieu proceeds to call neo-liberalism 'a fatalistic discourse' (1998: 55). The analysis of this discourse – the attempt to think through the circulation of power that subtends medical consumerism – may be the best antidote to that fatalism.

Acknowledgement

My thanks to this volume's editors and to Erik Parens for comments on an earlier draft. Mike Atkinson brought publication of *The Art of Cosmetic Beauty* to my attention, and Ron Epstein, MD, complicated a sociological analysis with singularly humane clinical experience.

Notes

1   A vague paranoia about liability leads me to designate physicians by a letter rather than their names, though these names are readily available by consulting *The Art of Cosmetic Beauty*.
2   As Simmel noted almost a century ago, 'Thus they imply that their best customers are the Best People – those who do not ask about prices' (1971: 183). The true pleasure of spending money often includes not having to ask how much.
3   Dermatologists Arthur and Loretta Pratt Balin (1997) present numerous and compelling testimonials to how their cosmetic interventions have improved the lives of their patients. Among sociological studies, Davis (1995) reports in-depth interviews in which women present their cosmetic surgeries as personal necessities. Bordo (1998) critiques the utility of these stories. For a discussion of the controversy between Davis and Bordo, see Frank (2000).
4   For an insightful critique of how such 'basic human needs' arguments fail with respect to medical services, see Silvers (1998).
5   Controversies over assisted suicide and the 'right to die' suggest that even the ultimately ontological value – life itself – is socially mediated as to the limits of its value.
6   Which patients allow themselves to be photographed, and in what terms they give consent, are separate issues. The present point is that my own utterly subjective scan of these images supports the findings of Davis (1995) that most women selecting cosmetic surgery seek not an ideal but rather what they define as normal. Thus, women were not as dissatisfied as Davis had expected with less than ideal surgical outcomes.
7   'When the vibrator emerged as an electromechanical medical instrument at the end of the nineteenth century, it evolved from previous massage technologies in response to the demand from physicians for more rapid and efficient physical therapies, particularly for hysteria. Massage to orgasm of female patients was a

staple of medical practice among some (but certainly not all) Western physicians from the time of Hyppocrates until the 1920s, and mechanizing this task significantly increased the number of patients a doctor could treat in a working day' (Maines 1999: 3). Maines also discusses clitoridectomy as a surgical intervention to prevent masturbation (1999: 5; see also 56–9).

8 The neo-liberal case is strengthened by the ambiguity noted above, that the same treatment serves diverse patient needs. Next to the MRI patient who waits anxiously to see whether cancer has spread may be a patient getting a scan to see how soon she or he can get back on the golf course. The problem is that the more discretionary use tends to trump in defining the public responsibility for offering the treatment, since clear lines between discretionary and necessary uses are difficult to draw.

9 Although cosmetic surgeons might consider Davis's data dated in terms of their current surgical practices, her observation is worth quoting: 'Nearly every woman I spoke with complained of some discomfort or side effects following her breast augmentation' (1995: 143).

References

The Art of Cosmetic Beauty (2000) Vol. 1, Summer + Fall. Dallas, Texas, US and Sydney, Australia.

Balin, A.K. and Balin, L.P. (1997) The Life of the Skin: What It Hides, What It Reveals, and How It Communicates, New York: Bantam.

Bauman, Z. (2000) Liquid Modernity, Cambridge, UK: Polity Press.

Beeson, D. and Doksum, T. (2001) 'Family values and resistance to genetic testing', in B. Hoffmaster (ed.) Bioethics in Social Context, Philadephia: Temple University Press.

Bishop, K. (2000a) 'Whose hands do you trust?', The Art of Cosmetic Beauty, 1, 84–8.

—— (2000b) 'Blue peel', The Art of Cosmetic Beauty, 1, 68–70.

Bishop, K. and Stapleton, A. (2000) 'Not all in vain', The Art of Cosmetic Beauty, 1, 98–100.

Bordo, S. (1998) 'Braveheart, babe, and the contemporary body', in E. Parens (ed.), Enhancing Human Traits: Ethical and Social Implications, Washington: Georgetown University Press.

Bourdieu, P. (1998) Acts of Resistance Against the Tyranny of the Market, R. Nice (trans.), New York: The New Press.

Buchanan, A., Brock, D.W. and Daniels, N. (2000) From Chance to Choice: Genetics and Social Justice, Cambridge, UK: Cambridge University Press.

Cox, S.M. (1999) 'It's not a secret but...'. Predictive testing and patterns of communication about genetic information in families at risk for Huntington's disease, unpublished doctoral dissertation, Department of Anthropology and Sociology, University of British Columbia.

Davis, K. (1995) Reshaping the Female Body, New York: Routledge.

Foucault, M. (1976) The History of Sexuality, Vol. I, New York: Vintage.

Frank, A.W. (2000) 'All the things which do not fit: Baudrillard and medical consumerism', Families, Systems and Health, 18: 205–16.

Grujovic, T. (2000) 'Editor's letter', The Art of Cosmetic Beauty, 1, 6.

Kramer, P.K. (2000) 'The valorization of sadness: alienation and the melancholic temperament', The Hastings Center Report, 30, 2: 13–18.

Leiss, W. (1976) *The Limits to Satisfaction: An Essay on the Problem of Needs and Commodities*, Toronto: University of Toronto Press.

Maines, R.P. (1999) *The Technology of Orgasm: "Hysteria," the Vibrator, and Women's Sexual Satisfaction*, Baltimore: Johns Hopkins University Press.

McCloskey, J. (2000) 'Web on', *The Art of Cosmetic Beauty*, 1: 30–5.

Muzik, V. (2000) 'Get under your skin', *The Art of Cosmetic Beauty*, 1: 64–6.

Parens, E. (ed.) (1998) *Enhancing Human Traits: Ethical and Social Implications*, Washington: Georgetown University Press.

Parens, E. and Asch, A. (1999) 'The disability rights critique of prenatal genetic testing', Special Supplement, *The Hastings Center Report*, 29, 5: S1–S22.

Schutz, A. (1971) *The Problem of Social Reality, Collected Papers I*, M. Natanson (ed. and intro.), The Hague: Martinus Nijhoff.

Sciolino, E. (2000) 'Iran's well-covered women remodel a part that shows', *The New York Times*, 22 September.

Sennett, R. (1998) *The Corrosion of Character: The Personal Consequences of Work in the New Capitalism*, New York: Norton.

Silvers, A. (1998) 'A fatal attraction to normalizing: treating disabilities as deviations from "species-typical" functioning', in E. Parens (ed.), *Enhancing Human Traits: Ethical and Social Implications*, Washington: Georgetown University Press.

Simmel, G. (1971) *On Individuality and Social Forms*, D. Levine (ed.), Chicago: University of Chicago Press.

Tauber, A.I. (1999) *Confessions of a Medical Man: An Essay in Popular Philosophy*, Cambridge, MA: MIT Press.

Veblen, T. ([1899] 1953) *The Theory of the Leisure Class*, New York: Mentor.

Weber, M. (1958) *From Max Weber*, H. Gerth and C.W. Mills (eds), New York: Oxford University Press.

Wernick, A. (1991) *Promotional Culture: Advertising, Ideology, and Symbolic Expression*, London: Sage.

Chapter 2

Fabricating 'health consumers' in health care politics

Rob Irvine

The category 'consumer' has developed through historical conditions to the point that it now features prominently not only within the sphere of private market relations but within wider areas of public life, from health, education, welfare, to law and politics. While the literature using this concept is well established, the 'health consumer' construct has provoked intense and conflicting responses. In contrast to the claim that modern patients act in the manner expected of market consumers (Haug and Lavin 1983; Sawyer *et al.* 1994) theorists such as Lash and Urry (1994: 207–10) draw attention to the practical, structural and ideological differences that differentiate public sector organizations from the private sector – differences which are said to make it logically impossible for patients to conduct themselves as consumers. This argument has found some support at the everyday level of social and political experience. In a study on the conduct of patients attending an Australian general practice, Peter Lloyd (1991) and his associates found that traditional consumer behaviour has neither solidified into a set of routine social practices nor been established as a new mode of reasoning. In the concrete world of living actors, it appears that people continue to think and act in a manner consonant with traditional models of patienthood. Thus, the concept is dismissed in some quarters because it fails to describe accurately the actual behaviour of patients in the concrete setting of the hospital, the clinic or the general practitioner's surgery.

But to fix 'the consumer' merely in terms of a set of behavioural traits against which actual behaviour can be assessed, reduces this complex term to a one-dimensional concept. Consumer discourse does not simply convey social experience, it plays a part in constituting social subjects, and relations between subjects. McKnight (1986) and Grace (1991) allude to this when they argue that the consumer imaginary[1] has been engineered through professional discourse and narrative, and then strategically deployed in a 'top down' fashion by the medical profession in an attempt to defuse grassroots resistance to medical power and authority. Following McKnight and Grace I propose to 'read' 'the consumer' as a historical product of social and political discourses. Unlike these writers I do not interpret the health consumer concept as the negation of political power and conflict; rather I treat it as a type of rationality that is integral to the exercise of power and instrumental to the operation of power relationships that shape the way things look and state what things mean.

This chapter explores ways in which the idea of the health consumer is used to subvert and modify relationships of power and authority in health care politics. The chapter is structured as follows. In an effort to see what the concept signifies, the next section maps the mobilization of 'the health consumer' within the discourses of resistance of social activists who contest the assumptions, meanings, values and practices of dominant professions and political agents. In order to analyse some of its reverberations, the following section probes the production of the health consumer concept within government policy documents. The final section argues that consumer advocates and government officials consciously and willingly subscribe to a common set of perceptions, judgements and values of what is acceptable, normal and moral consumer conduct. This shared ideology functions to reproduce existing relations of power and authority in health care institutions that ensure that patients are maintained in their position of subordination to health care providers.

The health consumer and the politics of resistance

The notion of the 'health consumer' materialized in public discourse in the late 1960s and 1970s, a period generally regarded as a time of considerable social, political and cultural volatility when progressive movements of citizens, intensely dissatisfied with their social status, promoted public resistance to major social institutions in a struggle for sovereignty and reform. This historical moment of heightened social strife extended to the health care sphere. Patient disaffection with public institutions and decision-making processes was impelled in no small part by the belief that service provision was dominated by self-referential professionals, inattentive or apathetic to the interests and preferences, both material and moral, of patients individually and collectively. Activists were equally sceptical of the institutions of government. Typified as a 'closed system', the health care bureaucracy was represented as an authoritarian and secretive social institution that was resistant to patient discourse and participation (Asher 1984; Bates and Linder-Pelz 1987). This emergent public resistance and opposition to the professions and public institutions has been described evocatively by Haug and Sussman (1969) as 'the revolt of clients'. It is against a background of declining social trust in and increased social antagonism towards the professions and the state that the consumer discourse, freighted with considerable symbolic power and rich in emotive and moral appeal, was strategically mobilized in attempts 'from below' to reshape medicine and bureaucracy. Critics of the system anticipated that once service delivery was 'consumer-focused' it would better serve the interests and needs of patients and citizens (Bates 1983).

In Australia, the first serious efforts consciously to inscribe the health consumer as a political concept in the symbolic realm of health care politics occurred in the early 1970s. The Australian Consumer Council and the Australian Federation of Consumer Organizations were among the first groups to put 'the health consumer' concept to work. In their 'war for position' with authorities the figure of the health consumer was the vehicle which consumer groups used to challenge power differentials. Thereafter, the consumer metaphor was mobilized as a central organizing principle and figure of speech by a range of more or less organized patient advocacy and user groups which sought greater social equality and democratic control of health care institutions (Carmody 1993; Grace 1994; Consumers' Health Forum 1987–1988: 1, 146). Fashioned by both cultural discourses and power structures, the political character of the project to encourage people to resist prevailing ideologies and professional privilege which foster their marginalization, is represented in texts and discussions of patient issues by the term 'consumerism' (Haug and Lavin 1983).

Why was the 'consumerization of discourse' (Fairclough 1994: 253) and the construction of a 'new' collective identity judged, if not necessary, then attractive? After all, 'the patient' represents neither a transcendental concept nor a timeless and transhistorical being. Rather it is a historical entity, a socially constructed and therefore malleable concept whose meaning has altered in response to changing social and cultural conditions (see Bynum 1994). Activists could simply have reconceptualized what it means to be a patient in late modern society in such a way as to demystify professional power and emphasize patient authority in a relationship between equals. I believe that the answer to this question is found in the symbolic world of representation and imagery, attitudes and practices which constitute the culture of medical politics. In particular the concept's embeddedness in professional regimes of power.

Professional discourses have had a dominant influence in consensus formation in modern Western societies. They have shaped the way things look and what they mean in such a way as to normalize and sustain structural hierarchies in the social reproduction of professional power and authority. From the nineteenth century the modern patient was formed within an elaborate web of authoritative professional discourse which delineated the boundaries of patient identity and gave patienthood meaning (Foucault 1977). In this pervasive system of professional representations, meanings and values, patients have been assigned a subordinate position in the production, negotiation and control of knowledge and practice. For most of the twentieth century, idealizations of the relationship between patients, health care providers and the state had conveyed an imagery of harmony and consensus which emphasized faith and trust between the key participants (Haug and Lavin 1983: 10; Betz and O'Connell 1983).

One can gain a sense of the tensions that professional ideologies provoked through the popular critical writings of Ivan Illich (1973), particularly his stylized representations of the laity's relationship with professionals. In Illich's writings, patients (along with students, social work clients and the users of other professional services) were typified as a social, cultural and political colonized population ensnared in relations of power which denied them an authoritative voice clinically and in policy-making. In order to facilitate change in the status of patients and displace professionals from the centre of meaning and the 'production' of health care, critics of the system argued that, for political reasons, it was necessary to redefine the patient as a 'health consumer'.

The construction of a new subject position, the health consumer, created new possibilities for people to imagine alternative ways of thinking and talking about lay–professional relationships which were fundamentally different from the disciplinary regimes of the past. Consumer discourse provided patients with a number of other alternative images and ideals for subjective orientation which encouraged people to think of themselves and their relationships with health care providers in new ways. The imagery of the health consumer in the market place emphasized not faith and trust in professional care-givers, but 'doubt and caution': health professionals were no longer constituted as disinterested experts dedicated to serving patient need, but as self-interested vendors of services, as untrustworthy as profit-making entrepreneurs. Health care workers could, therefore, be represented as legitimate objects of suspicion who posed, at least potentially, a threat to patients and their interests. Some of these points were raised by the prominent legal scholar and social commentator Ian Kennedy in his discussion of modern medicine. Kennedy (1981: 116–17) observed:

> Consumerism is better understood as being concerned with protecting what are judged, at the time, to be the legitimate interests of the consumer, in the face of the greater power of others to hurt or injure or exploit him [sic] or to undermine his power of self-determination and responsibility for his own destiny.

Health consumers, however, are not simply constituted within a language of resistance and opposition which systematically encourages people to imagine and represent themselves as something other than how health workers imagine them. With the advent of consumerism, there is another possibility, namely, that people may develop their own 'voice' and be creative in new ways, and thus forge an alternative identity from that of the traditional patient. A related purpose of consumer discourse is to foster a more socially and politically significant actor. This narrative, and its logic, leads inevitably to health consumers and their advocates claiming a share of power within a democratized social and cultural system of health care provision. Under the new regime, professionals were to lose their exclusive sovereign authority to develop, define and articulate the ethical, moral and material imperatives of medical care. As Kennedy points out, as the consumers of health care services, patients are assigned a certain power by being placed at the centre of action and by having their sovereignty given primacy, and not that of the professions. With their cognitive competence taken as given, health consumers are understood to be self-actualizing, self-activated, autonomous social agents who cannot be subordinated to the professionals, and are capable, with adequate information, of formulating their own intentions, deciding their own preferences and wants, and making rational choices about their fate. At the level of everyday experience, this imaginary is typified by the vast array of self-help manuals that have been published since the 1970s, such as the popular and influential *Our Bodies Ourselves* (Phillips and Rakusen 1978).

This 'new' vision of identity superimposed on the patient category is, in addition, clearly meant to influence patient subjectivity and identity, and be translated into new social and cultural practices and ways of thinking. Consumer groups and their advocates (consumerists) have issued a torrent of documents and rules which instruct the public about what they ought to think, feel and act and what they ought to value in their consumer persona (Bastion 1991; Consumers' Health Forum 1993). As health consumers, people are meant to develop new relations with health care providers, policy-makers and themselves. At the level of practical conduct they are admonished not to act unthinkingly and not to defer to the sovereign will of health care providers. Rather they are encouraged to seek out information, for example, finding out the side-effects of prescribed medicine, consult books for guidance on how to cope with illness, and investigate and evaluate the available medical services (Hibbard and Weeks 1987; Hugman 1994). They are also spurred on to engage in self-care and health-promoting behaviours (Grace 1991; Consumers' Health Forum 1993: 25–30).

Consumerism as a force has certainly registered on health care policy and practice, particularly in regard to information flows from health care institutions to patients. Yet despite the progressivist orientation, the new idealism that has been articulated within social movements of protest and resistance has been vulnerable to conservative appropriation and reinterpretation. In the next section I examine the production of the health consumer in institutional sites of production linked with the workings of official power of the administrative state.

The health consumer in the domain of government

In respect to political narrative, from the late 1970s through the 1980s the prevailing sentiment among Australian public officials and political agents to the ideology of consumerism seems to have been that of indifference and inaction (Sylvan 1994: 1; NCAAC 1992: 16), and not until the early 1990s do we witness an internal shift in the official discourses of the state. At this point the health consumer emerges as a recurring motif in the written and oral utterances of officials and political decision makers. Today, 'the health consumer' features prominently in a range of policy statements, policy directives, handbooks, information sheets, consumer rights statements and charters which issue from government and quasi-government instrumentalities and health facilities.[2]

A number of observers who have focused on the mobilizing aspects of consumerism argue that the state now seems to share with social activists a certain affinity for consumer ideology. References in official utterances to the health consumer as a pre-eminent form of identity is interpreted as a clear indication of the rhetorical power of the term and a measure of the success of an organized social movement of protest and resistance to have its preferred meanings and interests integrated within government policy and practice (Short 1998a, 1998b; Baldry 1993). We should not underestimate the possibilities for these connections. Impelled by humanistic considerations, it is conceivable that officials of the state have responded to patient demands to have their knowledge respected as an authoritative source of knowledge and to have their interests and desires count for something. Yet, nor should we take the connection between public protest and official discourse for granted by playing down or ignoring the capacity of officials of the administrative state to create the illusion that they have been sympathetic to patient interests by responding to their demands, while reproducing and maintaining existing differential power relations in society. In the process of garnering a consensus for their policies, officials and political agents take an active part in the construction of meanings, vocabularies and rationalities in the construction, justification and legitimation of public policy. To win ideological consent to rule, officials and political decision makers take up the language of the governed and appropriate progressive political ideas, strategically manipulating or altering them in order to produce a 'shared' framework that may be more apparent than real (Gramsci 1971: 323–5; Habermas 1984).

It is also important that we locate official consumer discourse in a broader policy context and in the material relations and conflicts that take place among groups. From the late 1960s through the last decades of the twentieth century, the policy landscape of Anglo-American countries has been dominated by concerns with restructuring the relations between the state, the professions and citizens (Hughes 1998). Within a regime of tight fiscal and monetary control, the discursive and practical realms of govern-

ment have been colonized by the controversial logic of 'economic rationalism' designed, among other things, to transform the social organization
of public sector organizations and reconstruct the culture of public institutions. Some of the more obvious effects of this regime include qualitative
shifts in public expenditure, deregulation, and the sell off, that is 'privatization', of public assets (Pusey 1991). Also of considerable significance to the
traditional professions of medicine and law is the reform in competition
policy. Another perceived solution to the problem of cost containment and
the new ethos of 'fiscal responsibility' is the complex and controversial
social logic defined as 'new management' or 'managerialism'. Inscribed with
principles and practices of efficiency, performance and productivity, this
model for organizational governance was originally developed in Japanese
and American private sector organizations. Concern over the growth of
public services and the regulation and control of expert service providers
impelled state administrations in Britain and Australia to import private
sector management regimes, complete with images of the market, and apply
them to public sector organizations in a concerted effort to remap the terrain
of professional–administrative relations and bureaucratic organization.

This new system of governmental rationality impacts on all levels of
health care culture and organization. Covering a broad set of laws, policies
and government actions it is materialized practically and in the thoughts
and utterances of officials and political agents as performance measure-
ment, quality assurance, care evaluation, clinical audit, clinical budgeting,
and case-mix. Managerialism cuts into and contests professional power and
authority by denying health care providers the professional autonomy that
they had at one time enjoyed. It is not surprising that in the early stages of
its deployment government authorities in the United States (Shortell *et al.*
1990), Britain (Hunter 1994; Cox 1991; Dent 1993) and Australia (Willis
1988; Sax 1990) confronted significant levels of professional resistance.
When new management systems and procedures were implemented, doctors
as political agents frequently diverted and diffused the effects of reform with
policy preferences that protected and extended their individual and collective freedoms and interests (Freidson 1986; Willis 1988).

My argument is that in this highly commodified social and political environment, government agents advance both practical and moral reasons for
policies which valorize the primacy and superiority of the market as the
institution for delivering health and welfare services. In the struggle with the
medical profession over programmes and schemas which jeopardize its
sovereignty, successive administrations found it expedient to creatively adapt
the health consumer imaginary to resolve some of the novel problems generated by managerialism (see, for example, Jones and May 1991). Consumer
rhetoric created a point for the managerialist discourse to penetrate professional authority. In order to reshape professional and organizational culture
and relationships, to make them compatible with their broad economic

vision, health officials link and align managerial and technocratic policy initiatives and the rhetoric of consumer interests, consumer demands and the satisfaction of consumer needs (Bastion 1991: 1; Health Issues Centre 1991). Put another way, at the level of everyday practice, the language of the health consumer is a vehicle which transports unpopular managerial reforms into health care institutions. It is also a useful instrument which legitimates the penetration of the state into the professional domain; through an appeal to higher principles of 'consumer interest', managerial incursions into the professional realm are imbued with moral significance.

To use Beck's (1986: 186) words (but in a different context), in tense struggles over hierarchy, agents of the state, like 'devilish' private sector business concerns, found it useful to 'sprinkle' the new system of governance 'with the holy water of public morality and put on a halo of concern for society'. There are significant interconnections between the popular visions of managerialism that are articulated both by officials and activists in their texts and discussions of issues related to professional regulation. Both groups also claim that their policy proposals are aligned to consumer interests (see Braithwaite 1993; Jones and May 1994: Keating 1990) – for example, the Australian Consumers' Association offered these remarks in support of new regimens which intensified and diversified the governance of the professions:

> National health service management standards are needed which incorporate principles of total quality management and best practice; monitoring quality of service, work place training programs, encouraging a team approach to workplace management and customer focus, including mechanisms to measure customer satisfaction.
>
> (Australian Consumer Council 1994b: 15)

It is worth noting parenthetically that in contestations with the state over policies which are perceived as antithetical to its interests, members of the medical profession have historically traded upon and appealed to the social and moral imaginary of the 'special qualities' of its relationship with 'their' patients (Hunter 1994: 15). For example, in 1995 the Australian Medical Association established a hospital hotline which solicited patient complaints about the care they or their relatives had received. The purpose of this exercise was to impede and, it was hoped, eliminate attempts by the state government to reallocate funds between hospitals and to gather information on the effects of managerial reform on the patient's experience of the hospital (*Sydney Morning Herald* 1995; 'Hotline for Health Concerns' 29 December p. 4). State officials appear to be playing the medical profession at its own game. The incorporation of the figure of the consumer in official speech means that officials can lay symbolic claim to being responsive to patient demands and aligning the state with health consumer interests. In these representations of the 'imagined relationship' between patients and the benign but active state, the state emerges from this discourse as hostile to paternalistic professional traditions and professional dominance of the health care system. Official consumer narratives convey the impression of officials and policy-makers as moral and ethical leaders who are 'in touch' with popular concerns and committed to the public will. Tendencies which are immanent in what Foucault has ironically described as the 'pastoral state' (Simmons 1995: 38).

The apparent alignment of official with consumerist discourse generated tremendous anxiety within the medical profession. Take, for example, the remarks of Professor David Pennington, former Dean of Medicine, University of Melbourne, about the dangers besetting the profession from without:

> When we see the intrusion of government into the very heart of professional functions, in seeking to regulate fees or standards or education or the organization of services, the picture (of the public image of and respect for the doctor in the modern society) looks even more bleak, and the growth of 'consumerism' completes the scenario of unremitting gloom which conspires to create a vision of the future filled with the deepest foreboding.
>
> (Pennington 1990: 242)

This is not an isolated evaluation. Similar complaints can be found elsewhere in the literature, voiced by those who are unwilling to accept the dislocation of professional privilege in a new social order (Broadbent 1992; Casanova 1990; Eve and Hodgkin 1997; Funnell 2001: 90–6).

In summary, the idea of the health consumer forms part of a general intellectual strategy that seeks to shape, and reshape, perceptions and definitions of what it means to be a health care provider. Formed from a range of ideas, attitudes and practices, the consumer imagery in official discourse can be understood as a politico-moral 'apparatus of capture' (Deleuze and Guattari 1987: 424ff). As a moralized discourse, the health consumer imaginary is linked to a process of consensus formation which seeks to influence and win the support of health care professionals for changes in the relationship between the state and the professions. Invoked within official discourse the figure of the health consumer forms part of a *raison d'être* which legitimizes managerial incursions into the professional sphere and the development of new disciplinary instruments for the collection and accumulation of information on, and knowledge of, the professional labour process.

Consumer discourse is a powerful and persuasive instrument which encourages people to resist prevailing ideologies and practices, and to form a new consensus. Yet the consumer imaginary embodies other, more conservative, ideas which emphasize cautious distrust of patients. In the section which follows I focus upon this apparent contradiction in consumer rhetoric which, on the one hand, limits patient choice and, on the other, reinforces a tradition of systematic professional dominance.

Taming consumer sovereignty

Peter Miller and Nikolas Rose (1997: 30) observe that in the context of the everyday processes of professional–patient interaction, the consumer is a 'highly problematic entity' which harbours a potential for disorder. 'The health consumer' is depicted within official and government discourse as a discrete, sovereign and autonomous *economic* unit, *homo economicus*; a figure which advances a view of patients as economically and socially self-interested agents. Health consumers engage with health care professionals as a formal equal. They also have the capacity to form, articulate and act on what they perceive to be their own best interests. Viewed from this angle, consumer discourse is both empowering and dangerous. Freed from the unifying power of sovereign professional authority, patients as consumers might contest the authority of professionals to prescribe knowledge and practice, and eclipse traditional systems of order and rule, at least theoretically, by engaging in personalized acts of choice geared to maximizing their interests and attaining what they desire. In short, health consumers may enact their 'autonomy' in exaggerated, arbitrary, self-interested and individualistic ways which disrupt the routines and 'cohesions' of the administrative order of the clinic and the hospital. Yet health care institutions, in common with other public institutions, depend upon stable and predictable relationships being formed between patients and care givers to get the work done.

Of course, public and private institutions anticipate this possibility and develop apparatuses of governance which discipline subjects, maintain order and manage the risk of patient 'non-compliance'. Bureaucratic rules, regulations, codes of practice and contracts serve this function by establishing the conditions and parameters for order in public and private institutions. For example, poor claimants who depend on the government for income support must satisfy a number of prescribed duties and obligations, such as undertaking and documenting job search activity tests, participating in programmes that prepare them for work, and so on, before receiving help. If they fail to submit to the department's rules and regulations, or if they refuse any job or miss an interview, social security personnel apply coercive measures, including stopping benefit payment. But patients stand in a different relationship to publicly provided services from other types of claimants. In countries which have a national health care system, such as Australia and Britain, entitlement and access to health care is not, *generally* speaking, made conditional on individuals fulfilling specific formal requirements. Nor do patients risk the same threat of *formal* coercive sanctions being applied if they either violate or fail to comply with medical or bureaucratic orders. In the context of these social relations, the additional 'strain' produced by the conceptual shift from passive patients to active consumers of health care products and services has brought forth other, interrelated, texts which limit the range of choices health consumers, as social agents, are able to make about how to conduct themselves in health care facilities.

Patients in the consumer persona confront a range of strategies and techniques which have been designed to undermine resistance and instil self-discipline. This system of governance relies, to a considerable extent, upon normative discourses which establish correct modes of thought and set the standards, boundaries and ground rules of acceptable and competent conduct – a conduct that is recognized by authorities as legitimate and reasonable. A commonplace and much favoured strategy in Australia, Britain and the United States is to specify various norms for conduct in a condensed form by embedding them in consumer rights statements (Department of Health 1991; Public Interest Advocacy Centre/Consumers' Health Forum 1990). The scope of this essay does not allow me to analyse in any depth the growth of 'patient rights talk' in the health care domain. It is sufficient to point out that the public is encouraged to believe that as health consumers they enjoy a range of rights. However, accompanying these rights, located somewhere between prescribed duties and freely adopted obligations, is a set of public responsibilities that are judged to be not merely expedient or useful, but a legitimate part of having 'rights'. Through the interconnection of rights and reciprocal responsibilities, health consumers are drawn into a network of power relations and techniques which channel conduct along socially acceptable paths.

The conception of the health consumer that is projected in rights discourse is that of *persona moralis*: an agent who has internalized certain specific values and practises self-discipline. Like other moralized discourses in the tradition of biblical morality, references to the responsibilities that health care consumers owe to health care providers and institutions embody principles disposed towards limiting, and in some circumstances eliminating, choice. As moral subjects, health consumers are meant to mediate self-interest and identify with others (for example, respect the rights of other patients and care givers). They are to take charge of their conduct by actively monitoring their behaviour for its acceptability and competence, to ensure that they use their autonomy 'correctly'. Patients as consumers have not, therefore, been conceded the right to fundamentally alter their relationship with health care authorities. Removed from the province of 'good' or 'responsible' conduct are independent actions which may interfere with or disrupt the rhythms and routines of the organization and the clinical and administrative order. [3]

There is nothing novel about authorities attempting to change the judgements, perceptions and prejudices of people, and shaping what reality is for people within a given culture. Nor is it new for authorities to attempt to influence people's self-awareness and images they hold of themselves, and give direction to how people should conduct themselves in relationship with others in public and in private settings. As Michel Foucault (1980; 1982) and Mitchell Dean (1995) observe, from the early modern period, the bureaucratic state and its officials have sought to influence public discourse on what it means to be a patient, a claimant or a citizen in ways which are consistent with bureaucratic imperatives. Therapeutic disciplines like medicine, psychology and social work have endeavoured to form and reform the capacities and attributes of the individual so that people comprehend and make sense of their respective selves and their situation in particular ways. Service providers exhort patients to 'behave properly', and to take care of themselves, their children and their relations (Parsons 1954; Cruikshank 1994; Culpitt 1992; Petersen 1997; Rose 1990).

The point being made here is that the critical arguments of consumer advocates do not necessarily represent a radical break from the past. In the name of good order, reason and fairness, consumer discourses appear to accept, and even approve of, traditional professional and administrative ideologies and practices. This condition of interconnectedness has coalesced around the theme of the social order of health care institutions. From this uneasy relationship, a dominant discourse has emerged which safeguards the rational organization of health care organizations and reinforces social relationships of inequality and asymmetry. We might infer from this relationship that the ideological power of the 'health consumer' metaphor does not stem from its role in challenging dominant ideologies, but rather in stabilizing and legitimating selected features of dominant ideologies. At the same time it masks, or conceals, its supporting function by means of moral lessons of patient 'self-control'.

Conclusion

In this exploration of the health consumer concept I have mapped some of its associations with health care politics and general shifts and trends in the regulation and rule of professional and lay populations. Under the particular historical and cultural conditions of the late twentieth century, 'the health consumer' has been formed through the operation of several discourses which target for change the cultural practices, values, attitudes, dispositions and personification of patients and health care providers. It is a force which questions the privileged status of health care providers and political agents and undermines the system which holds distinctions between professionals and knowledge experts, and the laity, in place. Constructed as a figure of resistance, it opens up some creative possibilities for the reform of patient relationships with the self and strengthens the hand of patients in their transactions with the medical profession and the state which might well produce the possibility of significant transformations.

Yet, on closer inspection, it seems that fundamental change to the order of things, notably the democratization of health care organizations, has not been forthcoming. Rather than marking a new or different subject position and a new political position from which institutions, such as the hospital, can be criticized and subverted, challenged and transformed, consumerism simply loosens the rules and expectations which constitute the traditional patient role. The idea of the health consumer takes on other forms and functions, which embody a potential not simply to transgress limits but to set limits and reimpose hierarchical relations in the health care system. In a period when 'fiscal restraint' and 'privatization' are the dominant discourses officials have used, the idea of the health consumer is a means to reposition the state in relation to health professions in a process of micro-economic and managerial reform. Consumer rhetoric has furnished officials with the discursive conditions, and a moral vocabulary, to intensify the scrutiny of health care institutions and professional practices and extend bureaucratic authority in the social, psychological and moral lives of self-regulating, but far from autonomous, professionals and patients.

Of course, any attempt to influence patient thought and action, and to govern populations, will never be entirely successful, particularly with such a contested entity as that of 'the consumer'. Ideologies, like the consumer ideology, are not immune to change. The tensions and contradictions which constitute consumer discourse may still offer new possibilities for people to resist governing discourses and to form a new consensus about what it means to be a patient.

Notes

1   I want to emphasise that because my aim is to tease out the ideological connections between the health consumer concept and political change, I use the concept of cultural imaginary in preference to that of 'image'. An image may be defined as 'a likeness or similitude of a person, animal or thing; a mental picture or representation; an idea or conception; an impression a public figure strives to create for the public' (*Macquarie Encyclopedic Dictionary* 1990: 463). The concept therefore tends to conceal the operation of underlying power relations. The concept of cultural imaginary on the other hand, when it is combined with politics, draws our attention to the active use of images, stereotypes, pictures, textual and visual metaphors, narratives and opinions which condition our thinking parameters and visions of the subject by actively giving our perceptions of individuals and things direction (Gilman 1995). Woven into the critique of the medical profession, the new cultural discourse of consumerism imagines medicine and medical practice as a source of risk and threat. And in a series of related imaginaries, the doctor is projected into the world as a 'misogynist', 'opponent', 'rival', 'antagonist' and so forth. These cultural imaginaries clear a path for changes in power relations between medicine and the public.

2   The extent to which this dynamic term has infiltrated medical discourse was

demonstrated to me as a member of a research ethics committee. The research protocol for the trial of a new therapy for the palliation of breast cancer referred to women who had participated in a focus group discussion as 'breast cancer consumers'.

3   For example, at the level of practical everyday conduct patients entering the John Hunter Hospital, Newcastle, New South Wales, Australia, are told to: 'Understand (their) treatment, its purposes and risks before (they) sign a consent form.' They are instructed to 'co-operate with the care and treatment offered'; 'answer questions about (their) health honestly and completely'; and 'keep appointments made for (them) or advise those concerned that (they) will not be attending'. Patients entering the hospital are also told what to value; they are to 'Understand (their) financial obligations to (their) treating doctor and the hospital' (John Hunter Hospital 1996).

References

Asher, A. (1984) 'Neglect of the consumer', in M. Tatchell (ed.) *Perspectives on Health Policy*, Canberra: Public Affairs Committee and Health Economics Research Unit, Australian National University.

Australian Consumers' Council (1994) *Australian Health Consumers' Charter: Draft for Comment*, Canberra: AGPS.

Baldry, E. (1993) *The development of the Health Consumer Movement and its effects on value changes and health policy in Australia*, unpublished PhD, Sydney: School of Health Services Management, University of New South Wales.

Bastion, H. (1991) *Making Health Care Better: Quality Assurance and Australian Health Care Services: A Policy Discussion Paper for Consumers*, Canberra: Consumers' Health Forum.

Bates, E. (1983) *Health Systems and Public Scrutiny: Australia, Britain and the United States*, Kent: Croom Helm.

Bates, E. and Linder-Pelz, S. (1987) *Health Care Issues*, Sydney: Allen & Unwin.

Beck, U. (1986) *Risk Society: Towards a New Modernity*, London: Sage Publications.

Betz, M. and O'Connell, L. (1983) 'Changing doctor–patient relationships and the rise of concern for accountability', *Social Problems*, 31, 1: 84–95.

Braithwaite, J. (1993) 'Identifying the elements in the Australian health service management revolution', *Australian Journal of Public Administration*, 52, 4: 417–30.

Broadbent, J., Laughlin, R. and Shearn, D. (1992) 'Recent financial and administrative changes in General Practice: an unhealthy intrusion into medical autonomy', *Financial Accountability and Management*, 8, 2: 129–48.

Burchell, D. (1995) 'The attributes of citizens: virtue, manners and the activity of citizenship', *Economy and Society*, 24, 4: 540–58.

Bynum, W.F. (1994) *Science and the Practice of Medicine in the Nineteenth Century*, Cambridge: Cambridge University Press.

Carmody, J. (1993) 'Healthy participation: a National Health Strategy background paper', in *Health Issues*, 35, June: 22–5.

Casanova, J.E. (1990) 'Status of quality assurance programs in American hospitals', *Medical Care*, 28: 1104–9.

Consumers' Health Forum (various) *Annual Review 1987–1988*, Canberra: Consumers' Health Forum.

—— (1993) *Guidelines for Consumer Representatives: Suggestions for Consumers or Community Representatives Working on Public Committees*, Canberra: Consumers' Health Forum of Australia Inc.

Cox, D. (1991) 'Health Service Management – a sociological view; Griffiths and the non-negotiated order of the hospital', in J. Gabe, M. Calnan and M. Bury (eds) *The Sociology of Health Services*, London: Routledge.

Cruikshank, B. (1994) 'The will to empower; technologies of citizenship and the war on poverty', *Socialist Review*, 23, 4: 29–56.

Culpitt, I. (1992) *Welfare and Citizenship: Beyond the Crisis of the Welfare State?*, London: Sage Publications.

Dean, M. (1994) 'A social structure of many souls: moral regulation, government and self formation', *Canadian Journal of Sociology*, 19, 2: 145–68.

—— (1995) 'Governing the unemployed self in an active society', *Economy and Society*, 24, 4: 559–83.

Deleuze, G. and Guattari, F. (1977) *Anti-Oedipus: capitalism and schizophrenia*, R. Hurley, M. Seem and H. R. Lane (trans.), Viking Press, New York

Dent, M. (1993) 'Professionalism, educated labour and the state: hospital medicine and the new managerialism', *The Sociological Review*, 41, 2: 244–73.

Department of Health (1991) *The Patient's Charter*, London: HMSO.

Eve, R. and Hodgkin, P. (1997) 'Professionalism and medicine', in J. Broadbent, M. Dietrich and J. Roberts (eds) *The End of Professions? The Restructuring of Professional Work*, London and New York: Routledge.

Fairclough, N. (1994) 'Conversationalization of public discourse and the authority of the consumer', in R. Keat, N. Whitely and N. Abercrombie (eds) *The Authority of the Consumer*, London and New York: Routledge.

Foucault, M. (1977) *Discipline and Punish*, London: Allen Lane.

—— (1980) *Power/Knowledge*, Brighton: Harvester Wheatsheaf.

—— (1982) 'The subject and power', in H.L. Dreyfus and P. Rabinow (eds) *Michel Foucault: Beyond Structuralism and Hermeneutics*, Brighton: Harvester Wheatsheaf.

Freidson, E. (1986) *Professional Powers: A Study of the Institutionalization of Formal Knowledge*, Chicago: University of Chicago Press.

Funnell, W. (2001) *Government by Fiat: The Retreat from Responsibility*, Sydney: University of New South Wales Press.

Gilman, S.L. (1995) *Health and Illness: Images of Difference*, London: Reaktion-Books.

Grace, V. (1991) 'The marketing of empowerment and the construction of the health consumer', *International Journal of Health Services*, 21, 2: 329–43.

—— (1994) 'What is a health consumer?', in C. Waddell and A.R. Petersen (eds) *Just Health: Inequality in Illness, Care and Prevention*, Melbourne: Churchill Livingstone.

Gramsci, A. (1971) *Selections from the Prizon Note Books*, New York: International Publishers.

Habermas, J. (1984) *The Theory of Communicative Action*, J. McCarthy (trans.), Boston: Beacon Press.

Haug, M. and Lavin, B. (1983) *Consumerism in Medicine: Challenging Physician Authority*, Beverly Hills: Sage Publications.

Haug, M. and Sussman (1969) 'Professional autonomy and the revolt of the client', *Social Problems*, 17, 2: 153–61.

Health Issues Centre (1991) *Our Better Health: Getting it Together*, Melbourne.

Hibbard, J.H. and Weeks, E.C. (1987) 'Consumerism in health care – prevalence and predictors', *Medical Care*, 25: 1019–32.

Hughes, G. (ed.) (1998) *Imagining Welfare Futures*, London and New York: Routledge.

Hugman, R. (1994) 'Consuming health and welfare', in R. Keat, N. Whitely and N. Abercrombie (eds) *The Authority of the Consumer*, London and New York: Routledge.

Hunt, A. (1999) *Governing Morals: A Social History of Moral Regulation*, Cambridge: Cambridge University Press.

Hunter, D. (1994) 'From tribalism to corporatism: the managerial challenge to medical dominance', in J. Gabe and G. Williams (eds) *Challenging Medicine*, London: Routledge.

Illich, I. (1973) 'The professions as a form of imperialism', *New Society*, 13 September: 633–5.

John Hunter Hospital (1996) *Information for Patients*, Newcastle, Australia.

Jones, A. and May, J. (1994) *Working in Human Service Organizations*, Melbourne: Longman Cheshire.

Keating, M. (1990) 'Managing for results in the public interest', *Australian Journal of Public Administration*, 49, 4: 387–98.

Kennedy, I. (1981) *The Unmasking of Medicine*, London: George Allen & Unwin.

Lasch, S. and Urry, J. (1994) *Economies of Signs and Space*, London: Sage Publications.

Lloyd, P., Lupton, D. and Donaldson, C. (1991) 'Consumerism in the health care setting', *Australian Journal of Public Health*, 15, 3: 194–201.

Macquarie Library (1991) *The Macquarie Encyclopedic Dictionary*, Macquarie University: NSW.

McKnight, J. (1986) 'Well-being: the new threshold on the old medicine', *Health Promotion*, 77–86.

Miller, P. and Rose, N. (1997) 'Mobilizing the consumer: assembling the subject of consumption', *Theory, Culture and Society*, 14, 1: 1–36.

National Consumer Affairs Advisory Council (1992) *How We Feel: A Consumer Prescription for the Health System*, Canberra: Australian Government Publishing Service.

Parker, M. and Dent, M. (1996) 'Managers, doctors and culture: changing an English health district', *Administration and Society*, 28, 3: 335–61.

Parsons, T. (1954/1939) *Essays in Sociological Theory* (revised edition), London: Free Press.

Pennington, D. (1990) 'Government and the professions', *Medical Journal of Australia*, 153, 3 September: 242–5.

Petersen, A. (1997) 'The new morality: public health and personal conduct', in C. O'Farrell (ed.) *Foucault: The Legacy*, Kelvin Grove: Queensland University of Technology.

Phillips, A. and Rakusen, J. (1978) *Our Bodies Our Selves: A Health Book by and for Women* (British edition), Harmondsworth: Penguin Books.

Potter, J. (1994) 'Consumerism and the public sector: how well does the coat fit?', in D. McKevitt and A. Lawson (eds) *Public Sector Management: Theory, Critique and Practice*, London: Sage.

Public Interest Advocacy Centre/Consumers' Health Forum (1990) *Legal Recognition and Protection of the Rights of Health Consumers*, Sydney.

Pusey, M. (1991) *Economic Rationalism in Canberra*, Cambridge: Cambridge University Press.

Rose, N. (1990) 'Government, authority and expertise in advanced liberalism', *Economy and Society*, 22, 3: 283–99.

Sawyer, M.G., Gannoni, A.F., Toogood, I.R., Antoniou, G. and Rice, M. (1994) 'Children with cancer: the use of alternative therapies by children with cancer', *Medical Journal of Australia*, 160, 21 March: 320–4.

Sax, S. (1990) *Health Care Choices and the Public Purse*, Sydney: Allen and Unwin.

Short, S. (1998a) 'Consumer reconstructions of medical knowledge in Australia', in A. Petersen and C. Waddell (eds) *Health Matters: A Sociology of Illness, Prevention and Care*, St Leonards: Allen & Unwin.

—— (1998b) 'Consumer activism in the health policy process: the case of the Consumers' Health Forum of Australia, 1987–96', in A. Yeatman (ed.) *Activism and the Policy Process*, St Leonards: Allen & Unwin.

Shortell, S., Morrison, E. and Freidman, B. (1990) *Strategic Choices for America's Hospitals*, New York: Jossey Bass.

Simons, J. (1995) *Foucault & the Political*, London and New York: Routledge.

Sylvan, L. (1994) 'Planning and the public's health: the consumer as silent partner', *Public Health Association Conference*, 29 September–2 October, Sydney.

Willis, E. (1988) 'Doctoring in Australia', *The Milbank Quarterly*, 66, 2: 167–81.

Winkler, F. (1987) 'Consumerism in health care: beyond the supermarket model', *Policy and Politics*, 15: 1–8.

Chapter 3

Health consumer groups and the national policy process

Judith Allsop, Rob Baggott and Kathryn Jones

Introduction

In the UK the role and influence of health consumer groups[1] in the national policy process has been little investigated. To date, most studies have either focused on particular conditions or on action at the local level. For example, there have been studies of voluntary groups for HIV/AIDS (Weeks *et al.* 1996), on disability campaigns (Campbell and Oliver 1996) and the role of mental health user groups (Barnes *et al.* 1996; Rogers and Pilgrim 1996). Two recent books discuss patients' groups in general. Hogg (1999) gives a descriptive account of recent policies to promote a more patient-centred health service drawing on her experience in the field. Wood (2000) has researched the activities of patients' groups in the US and the UK at local and national level using data from the groups themselves. Both authors conclude that the patient interest is weakly represented, although neither investigates how the collective representation of consumer interests is channelled through participation in the policy process, how political networks are established and utilized and how effective they are.

There is therefore a case for a more general assessment. In the UK, health consumer groups have been increasing in number and have become more diverse. Of particular interest is the growth of alliances between groups. Furthermore, governments, the professions and business are seeking to involve health service users in their decision-making and frequently draw on the membership of health consumer groups. This activity too requires investigation. In some countries – for example, in Holland (Dekkers 1997; Blaauwbroek 1998) and in Australia (Bastian 1998) – the health consumer and patients and carer organizations are represented through a central body with significant government funding. This is not yet the case in the UK although it may develop in the wake of the current NHS Plan (Department of Health 2000a).

In this chapter, the aim is to discuss a number of sociological and political theories that are relevant to analysing the role of health consumer groups and then to draw on the first stage of a research project funded by the Economic and Social Research Council (ESRC) which is currently in progress.[2] The aim of the research was to first investigate the ways in which such groups involve their membership in decision-making and, second, to identify the ways in which they participated in the policy-making process with government, Parliament and other professional and business interests. There were several underlying questions in the research:

*   Could health consumer groups be said to be a form of new social movement?
*   Do groups generate a form of 'social capital'?
*   Do health consumer groups represent a participatory form of democratic association?
*   Are there particular policy networks which are particularly effective in influencing policy?
*   How important is a specific policy context to explaining their success or lack of it?

In order to address these issues, the research concentrated on five disease and condition areas: namely, arthritis, cancer, heart and circulatory disease, maternity and childbirth, and mental health. These were chosen advisedly not merely to limit the scope of the research, but to reflect different illness conditions and life events as well as a variety of policy contexts.

For the first stage of the research reported here, a structured questionnaire was designed to provide descriptive statistics of the field and to illuminate key theoretical issues. At the time of writing, data from the second and third stage semi-structured interviews with a cross-section of groups and other stakeholders such as civil servants, politicians and professionals are being analysed.

Approaches to studying the policy process

Social movements and democratic theory

There has been considerable interest in what have been called the 'new social movements' (Habermas 1984; Offe 1985; Giddens 1994). The label of new social movements was initially used to describe the civil rights, gay and lesbian movements, environmental, women's, disability and HIV/AIDs movements which developed in the 1970s and 1980s. Such groups have often adopted unconventional strategies for protest. Byrne (1997) notes that the common feature of these social movements is that their adherents are motivated by expressive considerations. Members have fundamental fixed values and construct alternative realities through a common experience or perception. Thus a shared sense of identity develops. Taylor (1998) argues that social relations within groups provide a filter through which the individuals become aware of their own identities while at the same time identifying a sameness with those who share this difference. They are thus able to develop a group identity that promotes solidarity. However, given that each individual is a cluster of identities and that these may shift, unless structures are developed which foster cohesion, new social movements may be volatile. While the identity politics of health consumer groups may explain the emergence of such groups most – as voluntary, charitable organizations – are quite formally structured and strategies for political involvement have tended to be through conventional political channels in common with pressure groups in general (Baggott 1995).

Based on the Dutch experience, Dekkers (1997) suggests that there are a number of strands within patients' groups that can be applied to the UK context. One strand is the sense of identity based on a shared condition as described above. This may provide for self-help, advocacy or be channelled into campaigns to improve services. Another strand is the concern for patients' rights. A concern for autonomy, respect and an opportunity for choice has led many mental health and disability groups to demand services that normalize daily living. In the UK, a more recent theme has been the notion of the patient as an expert (Department of Health 1999). Many conditions require considerable self-management and patients become knowledgeable about their own condition and aware of the treatment choices available. Groups may be established to inform professionals and to raise public awareness. As a consequence of their diverse origins, health consumer groups pursue their goals in a variety of ways. Some provide services. Others promote self-help, or seek to raise awareness or campaign and many combine a range of activities.

In the UK, a recent development has been the growth of 'umbrella' groups – that is, of alliances between groups with a common interest. These are also various. Some share the experience of a similar condition. For example, the Long Term Medical Conditions Alliance now has over a hundred health consumer groups as members. As its name implies, it has a concern for those chronic conditions that affect daily living and where, perforce, the patient and the carer become experts. On the other hand, the Genetic Interest Group is made up of groups whose members have an inherited condition or who are carers for such people. Other alliances are based on an interest in policy change for a particular group. For example, the Maternity Alliance consists of trade unions and professional associations as well as maternity groups and is concerned with all aspects of maternity, from employment rights to childbirth. The recently established Mental Health Alliance consists of about 40 organizations covering health consumer groups, professional associations and research bodies. This is a loose coalition with a common interest in sharing information to lobby on proposed mental health legislation. The alliance contains groups with different views on the balance to be struck between individual rights and public safety. Of particular interest is the Patients' Forum, an alliance of about 60 national organizations, including health consumer groups and affiliated professional groups. The Forum was particularly active in gathering together the expertise necessary to obtain amendments to the 1999 NHS Bill and, in 2001, is promoting a national patients' organization to be funded, at least in part, by government.

The growth of participative politics

The growth of health consumer groups and alliances can be seen as a part of the growth of what some political scientists have referred to as a more participative, or associative, form of politics (Marr 1995; Hirst 1996). Marr refers to the growth of a community politics that seeks to mobilize marginal communities. He says:

> There is growing and irrefutable evidence of the rise of a new kind of community politics in Britain. There are community schools, urban villages, self-help groups of all kinds, neighbourhood patrols, housing co-operatives and associations, credit unions, local campaigning organizations, all of them meaning more to many middle and working class communities than traditional politics has realized.
>
> (Marr 1995: 100–1)

Such developments have been explained in various ways as stemming from the post-modern condition, which has led to a search for more meaningful forms of association and a rejection of conventional politics. For example, Habermas (1984) pointed to the failure of the 'instrumental rationality', which focuses on ends and goals and is the discourse of government and the expert, to connect with the experience or 'lifeworlds' of ordinary people. Dryzek (1990) similarly points to the dominance of instrumental action and the way in which the objectivist knowledge held by professionals, managers and experts is privileged and drives out the consideration of moral, aesthetic and experiential knowledge. Giddens (1994) notes the growing scepticism of political and professional elites and of the benefits of the drive for economic prosperity and of social and political reform. These fail to quiet the heightened awareness of uncertainty and risk in the health area, and although technologies continue to advance, new developments pose dilemmas as well as opportunities. Moreover, in the media there is a continuous trail of adverse events which underline the fallibility of expert systems.

One response to this uncertainty has been a call for a different form of participative politics. In terms of normative theory, there are also similarities between accounts of what constitutes a participative politics. For example, Habermas (1984) declares that there is a potential for a 'communicative rationality'. This, he suggests, can be achieved through the construction of democratic institutions that encourage the direct participation of individuals and the opportunity for dialogue. Within political science, Dryzek (1990) develops these arguments to provide an agenda for an emancipatory politics (see Sanderson 1999 for a commentary). This notion may be seen as utopian. It rests on the assumption, not only that there will be an opportunity for participation, but also that citizens will be willing to become involved in political decision-making; and that they should be capable of making arguments and questioning proposals put forward by others. Giddens (1994) uses the term 'deliberative democracy' to emphasize the central importance of dialogue in such notions. Participants reach a judgement on the basis of a debate and work to establish relations based on 'active trust'. The process is about achieving a resolution in which the implications for each party are understood. This can sometimes lead to more innovative decisions among participants who are seen as 'stakeholders' in a deliberative process rather than simply as people representing particular interests. In health consumer groups that are membership-based, and in alliances, it is likely that such processes would be attractive as they allow a collective view to emerge while still preserving group autonomy.

These ideas about the importance of trust and a shared understanding of different forms of knowledge can be linked to discussions within political science of the role of 'social capital' in building and strengthening civic society and its place in political renewal. Putnam (1995: 57), one of the main exponents, has stated that 'social capital' refers to the features of social organization such as networks, norms and social trust that facilitate coordination and cooperation for social benefit. His argument, based on a long-term research project on government in northern Italy, is that people learn to trust one another through interaction in associations and through informal social networks. The norms of trust and reciprocity can then be conveyed into the society at large and a capacity for collective action in relation to government institutions is thus created. He sees civic engagement and responsive government being locked together in a virtuous circle as opposed to a vicious circle of poor government, distrust and disorder (Putnam 1993: 117).

Putnam's work has been widely criticized (Foley and Edwards 1999). It has been argued that he neglects the impact of large-scale social and economic changes on the capacity for building social capital. Critics also challenge his view that the quality of governance is directly related to the quality of civil networks. Authors such as Coleman (1988) suggest that social capital is relational and therefore specific to particular relations and contexts. According to this view, a given form of social capital may facilitate certain actions but may have no effect upon, or even inhibit, others. A further criticism of Putnam's approach is that it neglects the roles of the state, political institutions and structures. As Maloney et al. (2000) argue, these considerations are crucial to the understanding of how social capital is created.

All these points are acknowledged in our study and we have an open mind about the ways in which relationships between health consumer groups may facilitate, or inhibit access to social resources that build social capital. We recognize that government structures play a role in shaping the contribution of these organizations. Furthermore, we are aware that the activities of health consumer groups and their relationships with each other and the state exist in a wider economic and social context.[3] Social capital is likely to be shaped by such factors, as well as by the increased knowledge and assertiveness of users and carers. However, it is also possible that the relational networks and resources generated by groups could be used negatively as far as the democratic process and the general public interest is concerned. Wood (2000) cites evidence of the feather-bedding of executives in the large US cancer research charities and points to poor accounting in some UK patients' groups. While we are not looking at funding issues specifically, there may be exclusionary practices as well as conflicts within, and between, groups that indicate the negative aspects of social capital. In our analysis, we will look for these as well as the positive aspects of trust and networking.

Bearing in mind these considerations, our initial findings, however, suggest that at the very least health consumer groups have great potential for building social capital. They are voluntary organizations, formed around issues of mutual concern. They have an ethos of consulting with their members, and can transmit these views and experiences to policy-makers. They engage actively with government institutions, other interest groups (such as professional associations and research charities) and participate in policy processes. Moreover, they have formed alliances with each other and draw considerable strength from such networks, enabling them to share knowledge and experiences, and limit conflict arising out of different aims and the perennial competition for funding and legitimacy, which is a feature of the voluntary sector.

Theories of the policy process

Theories of the policy process, which are concerned with how policies get made and implemented, are also of particular relevance to understanding the relationships between health consumer groups and the state. For example, what is the role of interest or pressure groups in setting the agenda and decision-making? In the health arena specifically, theorists have focused on the interplay of structural interests. Alford (1975) argued that state and medical interests were the dominant interests in health care while the community interest was repressed. Other analysts in the US and the UK have included the interests of capital as part of the state/industrial complex. This is said to drive, as well as inhibit, policy change (Moran 1999).

Some theorists such as Cawson (1985) analyse the governance of the NHS in the UK in terms of corporatism. Indeed, in an earlier account,

Klein (1977) referred to a 'concordat' between ministers, Department of Health civil servants and managers and the institutions of medicine. However, recent changes indicate a greater fluidity in structured interests. The corporatist concordat was tested by the Conservative government's health reforms of 1990 (Ham 2000). Subsequently, while 'normal politics' have been resumed in terms of consultation and deliberation between the profession and government, this is in the context of a clear agenda by the present Labour government to 'modernize' health care and involve patients more extensively in decision-making.

Also relevant to explaining how health consumer groups may or may not influence the policy process is the contribution of theorists who work within the paradigm of policy communities or policy networks. The notion of a policy community or policy network is an attempt to build a bridge between the micro level of individual actors within the policy process and macro level theories of corporate interests. Jordan (1981: 105) defined the term 'policy community' as: 'A comparatively small circle of participants that civil servants might define as being of relevance for any particular policy.' Subsequently, Marsh and Rhodes (1992) and Rhodes (1997) developed the term 'policy network' as a generic label which included a range of different state–group relationships. The authors identified two ideal types of policy networks and communities: stable and highly integrated and interdependent communities of organizations; and issue networks. The latter are looser collections of organizations exhibiting instability and a small degree of interdependence. They hypothesized that changes in the composition and nature of policy networks would have an impact on policy outputs.

Other approaches have focused on the importance of political resources, as well as other factors in shaping the relationship between groups and government. For example, Saward (1990) identifies six resources which groups might bring to the policy process: non-positional authority (skills, expertise and status), size, group cohesiveness, labour inputs and control of these, capital inputs and the salience of group values to the wider society. He suggests that medical professional organizations are high in these resources, in contrast to health consumer groups that are relatively weak as they rely on a narrow value set and may lack wider support. He argues:

> Small value based groups can be the sole suppliers of very particular value-sets, but in broad terms the lack of cohesiveness of such groups contributes to government being able to pick and choose among potential co-optees, according to which values they wish to associate themselves with.
>
> (Saward 1990: 595)

Using Saward's identification of different sorts of resource, it can be argued that these are not static. Although power may reside with government as the co-opter, the influence of a group may change as they gain in any of the resources. For instance, the acknowledgement of expertise or the development of greater cohesiveness, or indeed government's desire to find an alternative to the authority on which it previously relied, might change the dynamics of the interaction and the influence of a particular constituency.

Other theorists have tried to explain the influence of groups in terms of the strategies they adopt and other organizational factors. For example, in an applied study of the poverty lobby, Whiteley and Winyard (1987) developed a model based on group characteristics. They concluded that the most effective and influential groups were those which had an open strategy (they attempted to influence a range of policy actors) were promotional, were accepted by government and had a lobbying orientation. Grant (1995) distinguishes between insider groups (those regularly consulted by government and more influential) and outsider groups (those focusing on other channels such as the media that are less influential). More recent work on policy networks has acknowledged the importance of the specific historical context in analysing a particular network. Baumgartner and Jones (1993), in their study of policy-making in the United States, argue that at certain junctures it is possible for those who are excluded from such networks to challenge the prevailing institutional arrangements governing access. Policy monopolies can thus be challenged and superseded. To be successful, excluded interests must create new policy images that facilitate the use of their perceptions, definitions and resources and thus legitimize their involvement in policy-making. Moreover, these groups may achieve both policy and institutional change by shifting policy-making into new decision arenas where they already exert influence. Once change is effected, this tends to have a long-lasting impact on policy as the new institution becomes entrenched. This fits with Kingdon's (1984) notion of the policy window when particular interests can begin to influence the policy agenda. He suggests that this occurs when problem streams, policy streams and political streams are brought together.

Clearly, the norms, values and assumptive worlds of policy-makers also affect who is involved in the policy process and how effective they are. Jenkins-Smith and Sabatier (1993) seek to explore this through explicitly linking values and beliefs to advocacy coalitions within policy systems. Advocacy coalitions are made up of actors who share a set of normative and causal beliefs and who often act in concert. They argue that these, along with government policies, are stable over relatively long periods. Changes tend to come about as a result of external factors, such as economic or environmental problems or technological innovation. These create a challenge to the old order and provide a space for the recasting of policy issues and the entry of new groups.

The development of a responsive public policy

Since the 1990s efforts to involve service users and citizens in general has been a recurring policy theme. Under Conservative governments, the focus was on the individual citizen. Generalized rights and performance standards were spelt out in charters for each public service. In the Department of Health, this took the form of a Patient's Charter, which set out particular service standards and the setting up of the Quality and Consumer Branch in the NHS Executive. In 1992, *Local Voices* (NHS Executive 1992) encouraged local health authorities to involve patients and carers in developing local services. This became national policy through the Patient Partnership Strategy in 1996 (NHS Executive 1996).

Under the Labour government of Tony Blair, the Department of Health has introduced a number of initiatives to obtain the views of the public through surveys, focus groups, citizen juries, citizens' panels and deliberative opinion polls. Like previous governments, the emphasis has been on connecting with individual citizens. The rhetoric of government papers stresses the importance of a new partnership with patients at various levels within the health service.[4] However, the NHS Plan for modernizing the NHS (Department of Health 2000a) is an attempt to embed a more democratic process into the NHS at a local level as there is to be scrutiny by local authorities. Patients' forums and patients' councils composed of local people will monitor and review local services. They will also make nominations to the trust boards. A patient advocacy liaison service will be established in every trust and health authority to support patients and enable them to voice their concerns. However, in England, the Community Health Councils that were set up in 1974 and have been the patients' watchdog, are to be abolished. Their national organization – the Association of Community Health Councils in England and Wales – will therefore cease to exist.[5]

Although less well publicized, the process for drawing up the National Plan has involved leading members of health consumer groups as members of the six modernization action teams. They are also represented on the NHS Modernization Board and the various taskforces created to oversee the implementation phase. This follows a pattern set by the working groups which drew up the National Strategic Frameworks (NSFs) to implement the government's health priorities (Department of Health 1998). So far, NSFs have been published for cancer, coronary heart disease, mental health and paediatric intensive care, and those for diabetes and older people will follow shortly. Many health consumer groups consulted with their membership as the guidelines developed, thus widening and deepening the consultation process. New institutions such as the Commission for Health Improvement and the National Institute for Clinical Excellence include lay members and are also a focus for lobbying by health consumer groups. In many respects, therefore, the government is creating the conditions for the increased influence of health consumer groups.

Health consumer groups: initial research findings

In the light of changes in government consultation processes, our research on health consumer groups proved to be timely. In this section selected first-stage results and some preliminary comments based on the second-phase interviews are presented.

In setting up the project, we faced a number of key conceptual and methodological problems. Hogg (1999) and Wood (2000) had used the term *patients' groups* but we rejected this in favour of health consumer groups as a broader and more comprehensive term. There has been a reluctance to adopt this terminology in the UK, although it is used in other countries, notably Holland and Australia, where health consumer interests are represented through the Dutch Federation of Patient and Consumer Organizations and the Australian Consumers' Health Forum respectively. The working definition we adopted was: a health consumer group is a voluntary sector organization that is concerned with promoting and/or representing the interests of users and/or carers in the health arena at national level.

The next stage was to identify the groups in the condition areas we wished to survey. As no single database existed, this posed a considerable challenge, and a variety of sources were used. A list of inclusion and exclusion criteria was developed. The general inclusion criterion was a judgement about whether the organization promoted and represented the interests of health care consumers. This covered single issue groups; cross-issue groups that had a brief including health (such as Help the Aged); generic patients' groups (such as the Patients' Association) as well as groups based on alliances. Medical research charities, professional and occupational associations, general disability groups, organizations that only provided telephone helplines, or were statutory bodies and general consumer organizations, were excluded. However, some of these were interviewed in stage three as stakeholders.

In all 186 groups were identified and in late 1999 a structured questionnaire was sent out to obtain data on the size and characteristics of groups; their activity in terms of their policy aims and interaction with government; and the barriers and facilitating factors to participating in this way. The survey achieved a 66 per cent response rate.

Most of the health consumer groups (66 per cent) were of fairly recent origin having been formed since 1981 and almost all (91 per cent) had charitable status. Well over half (61 per cent) covered the whole of the UK including Northern Ireland. They could thus claim to draw on a wide range of experiences across the country and within different administrations. About one-fifth stated that they also supported health care users overseas. Some had links with international bodies, while a few claimed that theirs was the only organization addressing the particular condition world wide.

The groups varied considerably in terms of income. While the majority had an annual income that ranged between £10,001 and £100,000 (38 per cent), almost as many said their income was between £100,001 and £1,000,000 (33 per cent). However, six groups reported an income of over £10 million per annum while a significant minority (16 per cent) had an income of less than £10,000. When the groups were asked to list their sources of income for 1998/9, membership fees and public donations were the major sources of income for two-thirds of the groups. Almost half of the groups (42 per cent) received funding from other charities and just over one-quarter from the National Lottery. One-third had grants from a source within central government, and only one-fifth (19 per cent) had obtained a grant from the Department of Health. Department of Health grants are mainly short term (three years) and are given on a competitive basis for specific projects awarded under the Section 64 scheme.[6] Interview data indicate that maintaining an income flow is a major source of concern for many groups and uncertainty can inhibit development plans.

Almost all of the groups surveyed (91 per cent) had some form of membership. For most, this included individual members, patients, carers and relatives. Two-thirds of the groups (68 per cent) had individual health care professionals and one-third of groups had professional associations as members. Groups that did not have a membership often employed health service users. Groups varied in size, although the majority were small, or very small. About half (56 per cent) had a membership of less than 1,000. A sizeable minority (15 per cent) of the sample had a membership of less than 100. At the other end of the spectrum, a few groups (5 per cent) had a membership of over 10,000. Some smaller organizations were run from the founder's 'front room', while many larger organizations had a countrywide network of branches, as in the case of Arthritis Care and the National Childbirth Trust. Almost all groups (91 per cent) maintained contact with their membership through a newsletter. Most provided information booklets (86 per cent), had a helpline (80 per cent) and a web site (70 per cent). These were for members and the general public.

Not surprisingly, given their membership base, our findings indicate a high level of involvement by patients and/or carers on the decision-making bodies of health consumer groups. Sixty five per cent included patients or carers, and health professionals were also extensively involved. Doctors were represented on the decision-making body of almost half of the groups although they did not always have voting rights. It is interesting to note that some groups deliberately chose not to include doctors for ideological reasons. Others did not do so because the issue that they promoted did not involve medical practitioners in service delivery. From the professional perspective, our interviews show that many professional bodies draw on 'patients' representatives' or 'consumers' for committee membership, and that they look to health consumer groups for 'expertise'.

In our questionnaire, we asked respondents whether they had formed alliances, either formal or informal with other health consumer groups. A very high proportion (85 per cent) said they had. The interview data provided detailed information on these alliances. For example, relationships between maternity and childbirth groups have been in place for at least a decade as there was a major policy initiative in the 1990s.

We were interested in identifying the range of activities undertaken by health consumer groups, and respondents were asked to rank in order of importance, 14 different activities.[7] The majority of respondents ranked the following as important or very important: providing information (98 per cent), raising public awareness (98 per cent), providing advice and support (96 per cent), promoting self help (84 per cent), fund raising (84 per cent), building networks (84 per cent) and influencing national policy (82 per cent). Groups were also asked whether their primary purpose was to provide services or to influence policy. Almost half (48 per cent) said their primary purpose was the provision of services; 16 per cent said their main aim was to influence policy while just over one-fifth (26 per cent) had an equal commitment to both. The remainder (10 per cent) indicated neither.

With respect to their relationships with government, most groups (61 per cent) thought that opportunities had increased over the past three years. There were interesting differences between groups within different policy areas. More cancer (71 per cent), mental health (67 per cent), umbrella (65 per cent) and heart and circulatory disease (60 per cent) groups than maternity and childbirth (46 per cent), and arthritis (33 per cent) groups thought that opportunities had increased. This matches shifts in policy priorities in the UK. In *Our Healthier Nation* (Department of Health 1998), cancer and heart disease were identified as major causes of death, while mental illness was a major cause of morbidity. There has been no similar focus on maternity and childbirth or arthritis. It would appear that the opportunities to influence policy are related to government priorities and that, to some extent at least, the agendas of groups must coincide with government to effect change. Nonetheless, the greater willingness of government to bring health consumer groups into the policy process suggests that a challenge to existing institutional arrangements (described by Baumgartner and Jones) may be underway.

We also asked questionnaire respondents to say how often they had been in contact with civil servants and politicians. This provides a measure of the breadth and depth of involvement. Three quarters of respondents (75 per cent) said their organization had been in contact with central government over policy issues within the last three years. However, their organization was more likely to have initiated the contact than vice versa. Almost half of the respondents (42 per cent) said that they had initiated the contacts while just over one-fifth (21 per cent) said they had responded to requests. Although this will have to be tested against the interview data, the finding suggests that the Department of Health has in the past played a responsive rather than an active role. The people within government contacted most frequently were Department of Health (DOH) civil servants (compared to staff in the Prime Minister's Office, Department of Health ministers and other ministers). Nearly half the groups (48 per cent) said they had at least quarterly contact with DOH civil servants. However, contact was almost as frequent with MPs and peers (45 per cent). The finding indicates that health consumer groups also use parliamentary channels. The media are also used extensively with over three-quarters of the groups (77 per cent) reporting at least quarterly contact. Umbrella groups and cross-issue groups had the highest level of contact of all, with over three-quarters in contact with civil servants at least quarterly. In contrast, about a third of the groups said they had no contact with DOH civil servants and ministers or with MPs and peers. This suggests the existence of 'insider' and 'outsider' groups.

We were also interested in what health consumer groups saw as their strengths in terms of their ability to influence policy. Almost all the health consumer groups (99 per cent) thought that their expertise on key issues and their ability to speak for users and carers were their most important strengths. Most said that their public profile (87 per cent), their campaigning skills (77 per cent), their links with the media (74 per cent) and central government (72 per cent) and their alliances with other organizations (76 per cent) were important or very important. Respondents said that the main barriers to effective participation were the lack of resources in terms of staffing (83 per cent), finance (80 per cent) and political contacts (75 per cent) as well as the lack of prior consultation (71 per cent). The other barriers which over half of the groups said were important or very important were the lack of support from government for the group's policy agenda (65 per cent) and their own lack of knowledge of the policy process (55 per cent). Our interviews so far suggest that some of the smaller groups, while high on passion and commitment, have very little knowledge of the policy process.

Discussion and conclusion

In this chapter, we have outlined the theories on which we drew to design our research instruments and provided selected findings from the questionnaire and the preliminary analysis of the interviews with the leaders of health consumer groups. To date our findings indicate that health consumer groups are an important part of health care delivery and that their membership and their role, in terms of internal and external relations, is growing. These groups share some characteristics with other social movements. They provide their members with information about their condition, treatment and services. They give opportunities for social interaction, provide support and help to forge a positive identity through enhancing autonomy and individual capacity. Collectively, groups hold knowledge and expertise, and members communicate with each other and the leadership through both conventional and Internet media.

However, health consumer groups differ from new social movements in two important respects. First, they are extremely diverse on almost every measure, such as objectives, interests, size, structure, strategy, tactics and the degree of stability. Although there are signs of increasing cohesion within certain groupings and an alliance of alliances through the Patients' Forum, this is far from being a 'patients' movement'. In the absence of a national patients' body, interests are currently too diverse to affect the government's agendas. The second difference between health consumer groups and new social movements can be seen in their tactics. On the whole, in terms of their external relations, health consumer groups have tended to use conventional and planned lobbying and campaigning tactics, not demonstrations or spontaneous action. Moreover lobbying has related to relatively narrow issues of concern to their membership. Our interviews with health consumer groups themselves and with stakeholders, such as civil servants, professional associations and business, have shown extensive networking and collaboration. But this is largely hidden and publicized only to the membership. The issues of concern to members are often specific, such as extending the knowledge of general practitioners about rare diseases; lobbying the Department of Health to fund new medicines such as the taxanes for cancer treatment; or contributing to service guidelines for mental health or cancer care.

On the basis of our findings so far, we would argue that health consumer groups help to produce social capital in terms of generating resources and building networks and relationships. These contribute to the democratic process in health care. Such groups have knowledge and expertise based on the experience of their membership. They have an ethos of involvement and, as our interviews are showing, mechanisms, which involve the grass-roots membership. Like other voluntary groups, they can be innovative, flexible and may generate considerable financial and political resources. The longevity of some groups, the development of alliances and the growing membership suggests trust, extensive networking and collaboration between groups – as well as between stakeholders. These processes reflect the characteristics of a deliberative or associative democracy referred to by Dryzek (1990) and Hirst (1996). There are some negative examples in terms of the absence of ethnic minority participation as well as of the decline of some groups and the splintering of others. However, the data requires further analysis to reach firm conclusions.

It is also clear that health consumer groups are being involved much more in policy-making. Patient and carer representatives are now routinely involved on advisory, consultative and executive bodies that formulate and implement health policy. Groups also have a parliamentary presence and have sought to influence legislation with some success. Moreover, they are frequently in contact with the media in an effort to influence the health policy agenda. The stakeholder interviews show that civil servants and professional associations value the input from health consumer groups and, in particular instances, we have found that this made an important contribution to debate and decision-making. This may be partly because in the present social and political climate the consumer voice adds legitimacy to professional claims. However, this is only in part. The knowledge, expertise and links with the grass-roots are also sought because they provide a different perspective on what, and how, services should be provided. The groups themselves rate their expertise both in terms of their specialist knowledge and their ability to speak for patients and carers as important factors in influencing policy. This could be said to provide the currency of social capital.

In terms of the national policy process, health consumer groups are now viewed as legitimate stakeholders. They are heavily involved in policy networks that were formerly the exclusive terrain of professional (and in particular, medical) associations. As noted, they appear to have achieved this by bringing to the policy process an important resource – experiential knowledge, expertise and networks – that the government finds useful in the present context. This gives some tentative support for theories of the policy process, in particular those outlined by Saward (1990) regarding co-option, and Baumgartner and Jones (1993) concerning the entry of new groups. The resources of health consumer groups are now valued more highly and this has contributed to their increased involvement and, in certain instances, to altering the detail of policy. However, this is not to say that the traditionally dominant participants – notably the medical profession – are valued less, nor is it suggested that they no longer exert a powerful influence over agendas and policies. Indeed further analysis of our data will shed some light on the relative influence of professional and consumer interests.

A further point is that not all health consumer groups have become engaged to the same degree. As noted above, there appear to be different opportunities to participate according to the medical condition studied, which in turn seems to be related to government priorities. Furthermore, some groups are clearly less developed politically than others and this translates into different levels of engagement. This inequality within the world of health consumer groups is clearly significant and we intend to explore this in greater depth.

The analysis of the second- and third-phase interviews will allow us to test the hypotheses suggested by theoretical work, to develop typologies and to gain further insight into the aims, norms and values of health consumer groups. We will consider what they see as their areas of knowledge and expertise; how they consult with their membership; how they interact with each other, with health professions and with the government and their views of this process. We will also have data on the networks and coalitions that have developed in relation to particular policy issues and how groups themselves assess their impact, or lack of it, on the policy process. Further, we will be able to assess fully the views of other stakeholders: civil servants, professionals, business interests and MPs on the role and influence of health consumer groups.

A final discussion point is the role of government in assisting the growth of social capital through extending support to achieve a more structured and adequately funded national health consumer body. To date, financial support from central government has been limited and ad hoc. Many smaller groups are unstable unless they receive service contracts. These factors may inhibit organization building and continuity. Government may prefer a babble of many voices but this could block the development of a facilitative and supportive body which could ensure a greater role for the patient and carer in the politics of health.

Notes

1   See page 57 for an operational definition.
2   The research was funded by an ESRC grant (R000237888) and is being undertaken at De Montfort University, Department of Public Policy.
3   See Lowndes and Wilson (2000).
4   This has been referred to as the Brighton Rock approach. Candy sticks have a message throughout the length of the candy. By analogy, the patient should be foremost in every aspect of NHS policy and care.
5   In 2001, the Health and Social Care Bill is going through Parliament and is therefore subject to amendment.
6   These grants are provided to the voluntary sector, which covers both health and social care organizations that aim to further the government's objectives in health and social care (DOH 2000b: 3). In 2000–2001 the Department of Health awarded 579 grants to 373 voluntary organizations at a cost of £21 million (DOH 2000b: 14). Three types of grant can be awarded: core funding, capital grant and project grant.
7   The list of activities was drawn from the self-help and voluntary group literature.

References

Alford, R. (1975) *Health Care Politics*, Chicago: University of Chicago Press.
Baggott, R. (1995) *Pressure Groups Today*, Manchester: Manchester University Press.
Barnes, M., Harrison, S., Mort, M., Shardlow, R. and Wistow, G. (1996) 'Users, officials and citizens in health and social care', *Local Government Policy Making*, 22, 4: 8–17.
Bastian, H. (1998) 'Speaking up for ourselves', *International Journal of Technological Assessment in Health Care*, 14, 1: 3–23.
Baumgartner, F. and Jones, B. (1993) *Agendas and Instability in American Politics*, Chicago: University of Chicago Press.
Blaauwbroek, H.G. (1998) 'Patient organizations and patients' rights', in A. Schrijvers and D. Kodner (eds) *Health and Health Care in the Netherlands*, Maarssen, The Netherlands: Elsevier/De Tijdstoom.
Byrne, P. (1997) *Social Movements in Britain*, London: Routledge.

Campbell, J. and Oliver, M. (1996) *Disability Politics*, London: Routledge.

Cawson, A. (ed.) (1985) *Organised Interests and the State: Studies in Meso-Corporatism*, London: Sage.

Coleman, J. (1988) 'Social capital in the creation of human capital', *American Journal of Sociology*, 94, supplement: 95–120.

Dekkers, A.F.M. (1997) 'The experience of the Netherlands: the Dutch Federation of Patient and Consumer Organizations', in C. Kranich and J. Bochen (eds) *Patientenrechte und Patientenunterstützung in Europa*, Baden-Baden: Nomos verlagsgesellschaft (English translation from the author).

Department of Health (1998) *Our Healthier Nation*, London: HMSO.

—— (1999) *Expert Patients Taskforce Established*, London: Department of Health (Press Release: 1999/0695).

—— (2000a) *The NHS Plan: A Plan for Investment, A Plan for Reform*, London: HMSO (Cm 4818–1).

—— (2000b) Section 64 General Scheme of Grants. Application Forms and Notes of Guidance 2001/2002, London: Department of Health.

Dryzek, J. (1990) *Discursive Democracy: Politics, Policy and Political Science*, Cambridge: CUP.

Foley, M.W. and Edwards, B. (1999) 'Time to disinvest in social capital?', *Journal of Public Policy*, 19, 2: 141–73.

Giddens, A. (1994) *Beyond Left and Right: The Future of Radical Politics*, Oxford: Polity Press.

Grant, W. (1995) *Pressure Groups, Politics and Democracy in Britain*, Hemel Hempstead: Harvester.

Habermas, J. (1984) *The Theory of Communicative Action. Volume 1: Reason and the Rationalisation of Society*, Boston, Mass.: Beacon Press.

Ham, C. (2000) *The Politics of NHS Reform 1988–97: Metaphor or Reality*, London: King's Fund.

Hirst, P. (1996) *Associative Democracy: New Forms of Economic and Social Governance*, Cambridge: Polity Press.

Hogg, C. (1999) *Patients and Power: Health Policy from a User Perspective*, London: Sage.

Jenkins-Smith, H. and Sabatier, P. (1993) 'Evaluating the advocacy coalition framework', *Journal of Public Policy* 14, 2: 175–203.

Jordan, G. (1981) 'Iron triangles, woolly corporatism and elastic nets', *Journal of Public Policy*, 1, 1: 95–123.

Kingdon, J. (1984) *Agendas, Alternatives and Public Policy*, Boston, Mass.: Little Brown.

Klein, R. (1977) 'The corporate state, the health service and the professionals', *New Universities Quarterly*, 31, 2: 161–80.

Lowndes, V. and Wilson, D. (2000) 'Social capital and local governance: exploring the institutional design variable.' Paper for the *ECPR Associational Engagement and Democracy in Cities Workshop*. April 2000. Copenhagen.

Maloney, W., Smith, G. and Stoker, G. (2000) 'Social capital and urban governance: adding a more contextualised top-down perspective', *Political Studies*, 48: 802–20.

Marr, A. (1995) *Ruling Britannia: The Failure and Future of British Democracy*, Harmondsworth: Penguin.

Marsh, D. and Rhodes, R. (1992) *Policy Networks in British Government*, Oxford: Clarendon.

Moran, M. (1999) *Governing the Health Care System*, Manchester: Manchester University Press.

NHS Executive (1992) *Local Voices: The Views of Local People in Purchasing for Health*, London: NHS Management Executive.

—— (1996) *Patient Partnership Building a Collaborative Strategy*, Department of Health: Leeds.

Offe, C. (1985) 'New social movements: challenging the boundaries of institutional politics', *Social Research*, 52, 4: 818–68.

Putnam, R. (1993) *Making Democracy Work*, Princeton: Princeton University Press.

—— (1995) 'Bowling alone: America's declining social capital', *Journal of Democracy*, 6, 1: 65–78.

Rhodes, R. (1997) *Understanding Governance*, Buckingham: Open University Press.

Rogers, A. and Pilgrim, D. (1996) *Mental Health Policy in Britain*, London: Macmillan.

Sanderson, I. (1999) 'Participation and democracy renewal: from "instrumental" to "communicative rationality"?', *Policy and Politics*, 37, 1: 325–41.

Saward, M. (1990) 'Co-option and power: who gets what from formal incorporation', *Political Studies*, 38: 588–602.

Taylor, D. (1998) 'Social identity and social policy: engagements with postmodern theory', *Journal of Social Policy*, 27, 3: 329–50.

Weeks, J., Aggleton, P., McKevitt, C., Parkinson, K. and Laybourn, A. (1996) 'Community and contracts: tensions and dilemmas in the voluntary response to HIV and AIDS', *Policy Studies*, 17, 2: 107–17.

Whiteley, P.F. and Winyard, S.J. (1987) *Pressure for the Poor the Poverty Lobby and Policy Making*, London: Methuen & Co.

Wood, B. (2000) *Patient Power? The Politics of Patients Associations in Britain and America*, Buckinghamshire: OUP.

Chapter 4

From pastoral welfare state to consumer emancipation

The case of Nordic alcohol control

Pekka Sulkunen

Lifestyle regulation in the welfare state

Most welfare state research focuses on what Gøsta Esping-Andersen (1990) called 'decommodification' functions of the state – disconnecting part of the reproduction process from the labour market by state-managed and state-funded income transfers and public services. These secure a living for people who for various reasons are unable to support themselves by earning a wage or a salary. It has gone almost unnoticed that the welfare states have also been major moral projects that have regulated consumption and lifestyles in precise detail and with very concrete objectives for the promotion of the good and healthy life. This has been especially the case in the Nordic welfare states of Finland, Denmark, Iceland, Norway and Sweden. In these countries alcohol control has been the flagship of the state's concern for citizen's welfare and health. Drinking practices and the market for alcoholic beverages have been the object of strict regulation since the late nineteenth century, particularly in Finland, Iceland, Norway and Sweden.

Today the alcohol control systems oriented to promote citizens' welfare and health are being undermined by two factors. First, the adjustment of the Nordic countries to the European integration makes it increasingly difficult to maintain national market regulations. Secondly, the ethos of the consumer society – itself the achievement of the welfare state – undermines the legitimacy of the state's role in defining and promoting the good life and transfers the responsibility for health to individuals and their families and private networks.

This chapter will use alcohol control policy as a case to explain how the Nordic welfare states evolved to be what Michel Foucault (1987: 68–70) called 'pastoral' regimes of power, and how this regime gradually turned into modern government of populations and, finally, into neo-liberal regimes of the consumer society (Foucault 1991: 99). The pastoral authority 'knows' – on various grounds, often on the basis of scientific theory and research – the needs of its subjects, even better than the subjects themselves. The modern government of populations is concerned with rates, prevalence and consequences of risks behaviour rather than the happiness of individuals. The neo-liberal late twentieth century saw a gradual erosion of the state's legitimacy in controlling consumption and regulating lifestyles in all welfare states. At the end of the chapter it will be shown that this erosion results from recast roles of private desire and public inhibition to private inhibition and public desire. Consumers are seen as managers of themselves, making choices and accumulating their social and cultural capital. The neo-liberal shift in the Nordic tradition of alcohol control implies much more than simply less-regulated markets: it is an example of the early welfare theorists' dream come true: the subjects of the state have become sovereign, now as active agents and consumers rather than as members of the population that belongs to the political community.

The key factor explaining why alcohol policy has so prominent a place in the Nordic welfare state agenda has been the involvement of the working class in late nineteenth- and early twentieth-century temperance politics. In countries where the labour movement distanced itself early on from the temperance issue, such as England and Germany, alcohol control never became part of the welfare state agenda. In contrast, in the countries where the labour movement was both an important support for the welfare state and accepted that drinking is a threat to the working class, alcohol control remained among the instruments of the state to promote the good life and health for all.

From rigorous state control to (almost) free markets

The alcohol policies that developed in the Nordic welfare states in the early twentieth century have been a spectacular historical experiment of social control. A few years after the First World War, Finland, Iceland, Norway and Sweden established comprehensive state monopolies with exclusive rights to produce, to import, to wholesale and to retail all alcoholic beverages other than beer. Denmark took a different route and adopted a much more liberal market system but introduced high taxation to hold down consumption. In all Nordic countries advertisement for alcoholic beverages has been prohibited or strictly limited and the price level is very high compared to other European countries. In Finland, Norway and Sweden the availability of beer, wine and spirits has been regulated by the monopolies in the retail market and by a restrictive licensing and supervision policy on bars and restaurants. Traditionally, commercial profits from the alcohol trade to private enterprise have been eliminated, but revenues to the state from alcoholic beverages have been important. In addition, the states have been very active in promoting temperance and looking after alcoholics. Involuntary treatment has been common until recently.

Today the retail monopolies that have managed alcohol sales since the early decades of the twentieth century remain in place, but other functions of the monopoly systems have been opened to competition. The number of bars and restaurants licensed to sell alcohol has increased and their business hours have become less regulated. The retail monopolies have made greater efforts to change their image from that of a control institution to one of service. The tax levels are on a downward course, and many other details are making alcoholic beverages more comparable to other consumer items, in terms of image and availability.

Some of these adjustments are legal reactions to European integration and the overall deregulation of the economy (Holder *et al.* 1998). The traditional Nordic alcohol control systems are often seen as outdated relics inherited from a puritanical past, and their liberalization as an inevitable consequence of the detraditionalization of the liberal late modern society.

However, the connection between the Nordic alcohol control systems and the modernization of Nordic societies is not straightforward. The notion of liberalism has gone through many transformations and even in its advanced form involves several dimensions, not only the relationship between the market and the state (Rose 1999). The term 'liberalism' in alcohol policy is even more ambiguous and contradictory. The Nordic control systems them-selves have been formed on the basis of temperance ideology that was modern, progressive and originally liberal in the political sense. In the early part of the twentieth century when they were established, the objective of the alcohol control systems was to ensure progress towards a better society by trusting extensive responsibilities over individual life to the state. Since then the liberal discourses have contained a diversity of arguments that sometimes are and sometimes are not connected, and they certainly are not consistently associated with more general social or ideological doctrines. Only in one meaning has the evolution of the Nordic alcohol control systems been unambiguously towards liberalism: from an almost complete elimination of private profit-making in alcohol in the early twentieth century they now have become (almost) free markets.

The history of the Nordic alcohol control systems is a story of three waves of alcohol policy liberalism: *the first* in the immediate post-war years, *the second* in the 1960s and *the third* still ongoing wave since the 1980s. All these waves have changed the relationships between private life and the state – or more generally, the public domain. Although each time the result has been a new move towards a free market, the *arguments used to justify the moves have been different*, reflecting the changing structure and stability of the welfare state ethos as a whole. The waves represent three entirely different discursive universes about freedom: the first centred on policing desire, the second on managing the consequences of the desire, and the third, emancipation of the self in the 'free' consumer society.

Modernity and the origins of Nordic alcohol policy

Nation-building and the Nordic welfare state

The alcohol control systems in Norway, Sweden and Finland have been exceptionally long-standing and coherent but not unique in history. Retail monopolies, relatively high prices, controlled licensing and inspection systems, tight marketing regulations, stipulations restricting alcohol use in public places, serving and retail hours and publicly run educational campaigns – in various combinations and degrees of severity – have been among the instruments of national strategies to attack alcohol problems in the USA, Canada, New Zealand and Australia, and the United Kingdom, as well as in most countries of continental northern Europe. However, in Norway, Sweden and Finland they have formed a system of interrelated parts in the institutions of public administration, voluntary organizations and market agents.

The source of the central position and durability of the control systems in the Nordic countries has been that they have been constructed and gradually transformed as part of the democratic nation-building and modernization in the first part of the twentieth century. Their construction was connected to the Nordic welfare states, as part of their moral foundation. Alcohol has been understood as a drug, and has symbolized moral degradation, poverty and social disorder – the opposite of the ideals of civilization and self-responsible individual citizenship that the welfare state has stood for.

The legitimacy of the state as an educator and an apparatus of lifestyle control has not been based only on interest group negotiations and successful class coalitions. National consensus about the good modern life and the public interest in social order, progress and civilization has strengthened the state's functions as an instrument of lifestyle regulation. In the Nordic countries, the progressive populism that developed into social democracy saw the national state as its instrument and partner rather than a threat or an enemy, like its North American counterpart has done (Sulkunen *et al.* 2000: 7–14).

Temperance and the progressive social movements

The temperance movements that spread all over Western Europe and North America in the late nineteenth century were an ideal-typical case of the worldly asceticism that Max Weber in his classic essay *The Protestant Ethic and the Spirit of Capitalism* (1970) thought to be functional in generating the spirit of modern capitalism. The useless pleasures of intoxication and spending money and time on alcohol, and the immorality associated with drinking, especially in public drinking places, was the antipode of the accumulative ethos of entrepreneurial life.

The early nineteenth-century American temperance groups were led by the Calvinist ministry of New England. Religion and individual perfectionism went hand in hand. To be saved was evidenced through a change in personal life, and the man of spiritual conviction could be known by his habits (Gusfield 1963: 41, 45). Also in Britain the earliest temperance pursuits were born among the Calvinistic Methodists. In Wales the mid-nineteenth-century temperance movement was influenced by Welsh non-conformist theology that required the followers of Christ to be noble examples of self-denying abstinence from all excesses, in business and in pleasure. In eating, drinking, dressing and all things pertaining merely to this life they should be 'moderate and reserved' so that they give proof of their heavenly citizenship (Lambert 1983: 117–19). As the 'progressive' temperance movements' activity developed into a 'moral crusade' (Lambert 1983: 252; Gusfield 1963) they started a struggle for prohibition[1] – denying the right either to produce, to sell or to consume alcohol – for everybody and often especially for 'others'.

Most of the major social movements of the last century – representing all social classes, rural small-holders as well as the urban working class and the nationalist educated middle classes – have included strong temperance elements. Moreover, the woman's suffrage movement was closely linked to temperance groups in the USA (Gusfield 1963; Rose 1997) and in Britain (Harrison 1971; Dingle 1980), and American middle-class progressives considered prohibition to be an effective measure against big business and political corruption (Timberlake 1963: 121–4).

The entrepreneurial classes in Western European societies found it quite easy to amalgamate teetotalism into their own religious doctrines and their everyday practices as businesspeople and industrialists. Their interest was to discipline the rising working class for whom the public drinking places were venues of political agitation and causes of relaxed attitudes towards factory hours (Barrows 1991; Brennan 1989: 269–310; Dingle 1980: 18; Harrison 1971: 62; Lambert 1983; Magnusson 1985; Rosenzweig 1983: 95).

The rising nationalist middle classes – teachers, journalists, the clergy and civil servants (Gellner 1988: 62) – had their own stake in the cultural struggle. They needed the support and loyalty of the people for their nationalism, and they developed a romanticized image of the people for ingredients in their self-identity as the leading element in modern society. For them, temperance policy was a key strategy to combat misery and immorality, especially with respect to family life. This was particularly important for women, who were largely responsible for the new reform movements in all parts of the Western world.

Finally, the 'dangerous classes' – industrial workers and peasants – were in a situation where worldly asceticism acquired for them a meaning very different from that in entrepreneurial culture: not accumulation, but survival. The fight against the alcohol capitalists was an early form of class consciousness and organized political activity, including drinking strikes, street demonstrations and parliamentary action as soon as political platforms were opened to them (Gutzke 1989; Roberts 1984; Rosenzweig 1983; Sulkunen 1986).

National consensus

In the countries where they originated – namely, Wales, England and the east coast of the USA – the temperance movements gradually lost their progressive role to other movements and to party politics. In fact many of them were transitional organizations that channelled religious and moral energies into party politics (Harrison 1971: 31). In the process, the centrality of the temperance mission became reduced and the influence in society ebbed.

By the end of the century the British temperance movement had become the conservative element of 'Victorian' morality, in which it was believed that social ills result from individual weaknesses (Dingle 1980: 222–5; Shiman 1988). As a consequence, the movement alienated the working class to such a degree that after 1890 most British socialists considered the temperance movement to be directing the working man away from his proper interests rather than serving them (Harrison 1971: 397–403).

In the same way the American temperance movements increasingly adopted a defensive position in national policies. Following Richard Hofstadter (1955), Gusfield (1963) concludes that in the move from an assimilative to a coercive doctrine of reform, prohibitionist arguments gradually developed into a theory of conspiracy. It was believed that evil men in the big cities of the East manipulated currency, tariffs and the national policy to their advantage. The temperance movement identified itself with an underdog position to defend the people's right to self-government and justice. Also its nationalism turned inward and took a defensive position. As in Britain earlier, the prohibitionism became a single-issue movement, and its isolation from wider political concerns was inevitable although its core values of the home, the nation and individual citizenship were still the same as in the wider social fabric.

In contrast, the progressivism of the Nordic temperance movements led them to collaborate closely with the radical nationalistic peoples' parties, the peasants' parties and the labour movement (Fuglum 1995; Johansson 1992; Slagstad 1998; Sulkunen 1986). The close relationship of the temperance issue to progressive social movements has given the alcohol question a high priority on the Nordic welfare state agenda. Whatever their class background, motives and interests, the temperance groups were out for political and not just personal reform. Of particular importance is the fact that the socialist labour movements in Norway, Sweden and Finland were temperance-oriented in the early twentieth-century nation-building process, and large sections of them have remained so until the present day (Johansson 2000).

Political liberalism and alcohol control

It is one of the paradoxes of the alcohol question that liberal parties have often, and not only in the Nordic countries, supported the restrictive policy. Liberal parties in European politics have been part of the development of parliamentary nationalism (Sulkunen and Warpenius 2001) and they have emphasized political rights rather than the free market.

Conservative parties have had much more difficulty in adjusting their alcohol policy programmes to their overall ideological doctrine. Conservatism has been a free-market alternative to state-centred planning economy, and this ideology of freedom has carried over to social policy, particularly as regards market regulation, consumer policy and public services. Nordic Conservative parties have also been typical representatives of what Ernest Gellner (1988) called the nationalist new middle classes – teachers, the clergy and the intellectuals. The moral stamina required of nationalistic leaders has implied that also these parties have until quite recently had a strong temperance orientation. In the Nordic context the Conservative ambivalence about alcohol is accentuated by the nationalist middle-class tradition.

Left and right

The alcohol policy debate has become politicized as a left–right issue only since the 1970s. In 1974 the Finnish Social Democratic Party adopted an alcohol policy position paper, which aims at handing over all alcohol production and trade to the state, including beer imports. In contrast, the Conservatives went so far as to consider the government's proposal for an advertisement ban (1975) as part of a wider socialist attack against private enterprise in general.

In Sweden the elimination of private profit from the alcohol trade, especially from on-premises serving, has been a strong temperance tradition across party lines. The nationalization of breweries has been a standing social-democratic temperance policy but not a priority.[2] The most consistent advocates of market liberalism in the alcohol trade in Sweden and Norway have been the *Ny Demokrati* (New Democracy) and the *Fremskrittsparti* (Progressive Party) that represent extreme right parties with neo-liberal and anti-immigrant agendas. In Norway the *Sosialistisk Venstreparti* (Socialist Left) has made proposals to nationalize the breweries since 1973; but the social-democratic *Arbeiderparti* (Labour Party) has not argued strongly against private profits in the alcohol business. The Conservatives have been in a difficult position, representing both market liberalism and a lenient alcohol policy under pressure from the extreme right, while maintaining their credibility in the alcohol issue among the nationalistic and Christian population under pressure from the Venstre and *Kristelig Folkparti* (Christian People's Party) (Anttila and Sulkunen 2001).

The break in the original consensus on alcohol issues in the Nordic countries is not related to moral views concerning the vice of alcoholism or the pleasures of drinking. Even the definition of alcohol problems – most importantly related to health, public order and concerns about young persons' drinking – seem to be fundamentally similar across party lines. The new divergence on alcohol policy issues between the left and the right appears to be related not to alcohol at all but to consumerism and the free market. The socialist parties find it easier to sacrifice part of the consumers' freedom and the profit mechanism in order to fight alcoholism.

Policing desire

Individualism and self-control

Modernity was built into the very heart of the temperance ideology. Max Weber (1970) had stressed that in contrast to earlier forms of Christian asceticism the Protestant ethic demanded the rationalization of the whole of a person's life under the power of reason. Also temperance reformers, following John Locke, made the modern distinction between will and desire. As Harry Levine has argued, the disciplined will was seen as a reasonable regulator of the natural desires of humans, and alcohol was seen as a poison that destroyed, not only challenged, one's will, the most valued underpinning of human dignity. This distinction made it possible for the early American temperance movement to define alcohol abuse as an addiction that results from defective will destroyed by the demon rum (Levine 1978). The will was to be trained to master lower passions – hence, civilization required constant practice of self-discipline and education (Valverde 1998).

The moral foundation of the Nordic welfare state rests on similar conceptions of the self-controlling individual. In neo-liberal discourse the welfare state is often represented as a collectivism that undermines individual responsibility and sense of justice, achievement and merit. In reality, however, the credo of the Nordic welfare states when they were under construction just before and after the Second World War was very individualistic. The sense of modernity as a loss of traditional communities – municipal community, the church, and especially the paternalistic 'household' that included often several generations and the servants – was a key element especially in the Labour movements' and Socialist intellectuals' rhetoric. The universal school system, obligatory tax-based social insurance and pension schemes, and a public health and social service system were not only functional in terms of modernization (this explanation argument has been often offered by Marxists and de-commodification theorists). They were also explicitly intended to provide for individual freedom from pre-modern social bonds. For example, the celebrated doctrinal founders of Swedish social democracy, Alva and Gunnar Myrdal, declared in their famous book *The Crisis in the Population Question*:

> Our contemporary social order is built on the ability of self-determination, by giving citizens a collective right to self-government. And this not only in political terms: every person in our modern society stands alone more than ever. She has no longer an intimate, solidary narrow circle to rely on, like the family, the village or church. She must therefore be able to plan her conduct and have visions over her living possibilities as well as to make many more decisions with her own responsibility.
>
> (Myrdal and Myrdal 1935: 309)

Naturally good desires

One of the great paradoxes in modern societies in the early twentieth century was that while they stressed individuality and self-control they turned to state-centred solutions in producing them. Temperance movements wanted legal restrictions, even a total ban, on the production and sale of alcoholic beverages; the welfare theorists developed schemes for education, public services and income security that were operated centrally by the national state.

The first explanation of this paradox is that the construction of the welfare states, and in the Nordic case, the centralized alcohol control systems, coincided with and depended on the establishment and consolidation of the parliamentary political institutions of nation states. Parliamentary majorities could be seen to represent the national will, and as long as centralized policy was supported by electoral majority it could be interpreted as the will of the population as a whole. Modernity in this sense meant also normality.

The second explanation of the paradox is that the idea of free individual will was not arbitrary with regard to the desires that the will was expected to pursue and satisfy. Since the Enlightenment the modern project has set culture apart from nature so that order and progress is thought to result when the conscious will (culture) controls 'raw' (natural) desires. Temperance movements were important proponents of this dualistic view, but they made another distinction too, also adopted from Enlightenment philosophy: that between artificial, unnatural desires and necessary, truly authentic needs and wants of man. The American temperance leader Daniel Dorchester (1884: 2) wrote: 'The true philosopher discriminates between acquired desires and appetites, or vitiated, perverse, and inordinate impulses, and those which are normal, necessary, and beneficial.' The desire for alcohol was thought to be bad and inordinate *in itself*, not just because its satisfaction resulted in bad consequences. In contrast, abstinence was thought to be in harmony with the normal, necessary and beneficial desires that belong to the virtuous modern subjectivity.

American temperance rhetoric was particularly influenced by the Scottish tradition of natural philosophy – John Locke, David Hume and Adam Smith. As Michel Foucault (1970) has shown in *The Order of Things*, Enlightenment understood Nature as a complete order. This view was prominent in the Stoic roots of Adam Smith's philosophy of the natural cosmic harmony that dictates our moral sentiments concerning the just and reasonable as well as our aesthetic sentiments that determine our judgements of what is good and desirable (Raphael and Macfie 1984: 5–10). These sentiments are the 'viceregents of God within us' and they connect us to the natural order, ordained by an impersonal but almighty Deity. They supervise our actions and judgements, punishing us when we violate the harmony and rewarding us for thoughts and actions when we conform to it (Smith 1984: 161–70).

The idea of natural harmony had a special place in Adam Smith's social theory but it has been widely endorsed also in the early twentieth-century reformism, including that of the Nordic welfare state ideology. It was a human duty to understand the natural order and to conform to its requirements.[3] The individual will was considered free, and self-discipline in consumption and health behaviour was deemed necessary in the production of welfare. But the form of life that the welfare reformers had in mind was not arbitrary and left to the individuals' free choice. Among others, Alva and Gunnar Myrdal were very clear about the normative content of their social policy. Naturally good and rational desires were to be singled out and supported by state social policy, against corrupted and 'conventional habits':

> The positive task in social policy is to make clear what a person should rationally desire in terms of her own values, if she had improved knowledge. ... Bad habits must be straightened out. The unwise must be enlightened. The irresponsible must be aroused. There is plenty of room for a comprehensive, socially organized education of the entire nation.
>
> (Cited in Hirdman 1997: 66)

Ronny Ambjörnsson, the Swedish cultural historian, has identified a term that the Swedish temperance socialists used to describe their ideals about enlightened modern working-class life: *skötsamhet*. It contains the same elements as its British equivalent 'working-class respectability': cleanliness, orderliness, temperance and self-respect, even a sense of superiority. But the Swedish word (*sköta* = care for) implies also reliability and a sense of responsibility for others. The normative model was the heterosexual isolated nuclear family that was based on romantic and free love between man and wife (Ambjörnsson 1988). Unregulated sexuality, gambling and immediate satisfaction implied also unregulated and conflict-ridden social relationships, whereas individual abstinence represented a wider belief in progress and civilization, through *bildning*, the self-education of the working class.

The first liberal wave: the civilizing policy

The first wave of liberalism in Nordic alcohol policy in the mid-twentieth century was a prime example of the modern paradox of individual self-control and state-regulated consumption. The dominant idea was that since prohibitions did not seem to work, drinking behaviour should be civilized and brought under control. The civilizing discourse was liberal in the sense that it purported to replace the polarity of drinking versus abstinence by more nuanced images of alcohol use, inherited mostly from European, especially French, bourgeois culture. To achieve this, alcoholic beverages should be allowed in the legal market, but under strict supervision by state monopolies and other government control agencies. The main motivation of the policy was the fear of the drunken worker (Peltonen 1991). The *viina, renat* or *brennevin* (distilled white grain spirits) was the drink of intoxication, revolt and uproar as well as the cause of social misery, especially grave on the family and its welfare that depended on the man's reliability and sense of responsibility (*skötsamhet* in Swedish). It was believed that if working men would start to drink wine instead of spirits, the drinking pattern and the sociability around it would also become tamed according to the self-controlling bourgeois model.

In Sweden the prohibition was defeated in a referendum in 1922 by 51 per cent of votes against 49. Instead, the alcohol monopoly *Systembolaget* was established, and probably the most radical system of pastoral state control over private consumption ever known in the Western world was implemented. Each individual was allowed a monthly purchasing ration that was controlled by the state liquor store. The rations were different for women and men, and they varied according to social class. Problem drinkers were not allowed to buy any legal alcohol at all. The *Bratt System*, as it was called by the name of its designer Dr. Ivan Bratt, was intended to eliminate excessive and harmful drinking, but it was from the beginning opposed by the teetotallers. Rationing, in one form or another, has been the position of the alcohol liberals even after the Bratt System was repealed in 1955.

In Norway the wine policy had long roots as light wines were exempted from the Norwegian Prohibition, and as soon as the post-war scarcity had been sufficiently overcome, wine promotion policy was adopted to fight the curse of spirits drinking (Hamran and Myrvang 1988: 243).

The ideal of self-control and good manners was based on the democratic project of constituting universal citizenship; the problem was that the image of the ideal citizen was class-bound and consequently the control system was discriminating rather than universal. Serving regulations, selling practices and the individual controls exercised over problem drinkers were selective and unfair towards the working class and all women (Järvinen 1991; Peltonen 1991).

In Sweden the civilizing policy was particularly a problem. The Bratt System already had been criticized for its undemocratic and impractical distribution of rations according to sex, age and class (Nycander 1996: 137; Bruun et al. 1985: 96-7). This tradition continued in the individual purchasing control practices that replaced the individual rations. Presentation of a personal ID card was made obligatory at every purchase, and the monopoly was given legal rights to refuse sales to persons with known alcohol problems or who had been caught for illegal distilling or blackmarketing. The number of blacklisted people went up to almost 20,000. It was not possible to control for this at every purchase, and as the selection of those to be checked could not be acceptable on an arbitrary basis either, an objective electronic device was developed. A red lamp was lit randomly on top of the cash register at each purchase, and if the lamp was lit the clerk – then called *tjänsteman* (civil servant) – took the customer's ID card and checked it against the blacklist (Ragnarsson 1993: 62-4).

The red lamp machine symbolized the problematic balance that the Swedish control system has been struggling to achieve between normative regulation and the legal neutrality of the state towards self-controlling individual citizens who expect to be treated fairly and equally, disregarding gender, race and social class.

Management of consequences: governing the population

The second wave of alcohol policy liberalism

Social discrimination involved in the normative civilizing policy was one of the factors that led to its crisis in the 1960s in Norway and Finland. The ideal of self-control and good manners was based on the democratic project of constituting universal citizenship. The problem of civilizing policy, brought up by the temperance movements as well as other critics, was that the image of the ideal citizen was class-bound and consequently the control system was discriminating and elitist rather than universal. Serving regulations, selling practices and the individual controls exercised over problem drinkers were selective and unfair towards the working class, the rural population and all women (Sulkunen 2000).

The second wave of alcohol policy liberalism in Norway, Sweden and Finland occurred as a reaction to such injustices. It was part of a general upheaval against traditional moral values in the 1960s, when the post-war baby boom came of age, crowded the universities and began a visible public life in politics and the media. This was a period of rapid industrial and urban growth in all Western countries. The educational expansion prolonged the adolescent phase of the life-cycle. The social support systems of the welfare state were consolidated, making individuals increasingly independent of their families. The new liberal attitudes towards sexuality influenced contraception policies and led to new legislation on abortion and marriage. Finland was first to allow legal abortion on non-medical grounds in 1970; the other Nordic countries followed that practice over the next few years.

One solution to avoid discrimination was a more equal availability of beer through grocery stores and not only in the monopoly shops in Sweden and in Finland. The number of licences to sell alcoholic beverages increased, the regulations concerning business hours were simplified and liberalized, and even advertisements for alcohol were allowed (Sulkunen 2000).

The radical generation

The youth cultures throughout the world in the 1960s that culminated in the student uprisings in 1968 were a generational break with bourgeois or middle-class morality, focused on the pleasures of sex, art and intoxication (Roszak 1968). Daniel Bell (1976) and Colin Campbell (1987) have argued that the radicalism of the 1960s was a resuscitation of the romantic spirit that has always been inherent in modernity. Alcohol consumption increased throughout the Western world, also in the Nordic countries. In literary and artistic circles sexuality and drinking became common themes of public debate, even provocation. The work of Henry Miller was popular among the young cultural radicals, as well as that of Jack Kerouac and Allen Ginsberg.

However, the reforms of the second liberal wave were very little influenced by romantic arguments. At least as regards alcohol policy, the Nordic 1968 was a solemn affair. In Finland even the political students' organizations were concerned about the equality of citizens and the consequences of drinking patterns rather than being interested in liberating the natural desires of human beings. The call for universal and equal citizenship in access to alcohol was the dominant argument.

The most important policy issue concerned the handling of alcoholics and other deviants. Involuntary treatment of alcoholics in institutions was specifically criticized by legal experts and social scientists in articles that led to the organization of The November Movement (Marraskuun liike) in 1967; with similar aims and purposes as KRUM in Sweden and KROM in Norway. This Nordic protest movement led in due course to both legislative reforms and changes in the treatment structures themselves (Hauge 1998: 228–32; Nycander 1996: 245–72; Stenius 1999: 84–101).

The population model

Although civilization and the constitution of self-controlling individual citizenship with equality of rights and duties was an important part also in the radical discourse of the 1960s, its content was the opposite to the earlier, pastoral regime of the civilizing welfare state. Now the Enlightenment idea of natural desires had disappeared from the public policy agenda. The welfare state – and equally the alcohol control policy – was said not to 'promote the good life but to prevent bad circumstances' (Allardt 1998). Bad circumstances would include poverty and exclusion, ill health and lack of necessary social and medical services.

In alcohol policy this implied focusing not on individuals, and not even on drinking, but on its consequences. Even the medium beer reform of the 1960s – making beer available in grocery stores – was seldom justified in terms of the pleasure of drinking. Its declared intentions were, first, equality and, second, an attempt to replace the strong vodka with the milder beer and in this way make drinking less violent and harmful (Sulkunen 2000).

Consumption increases that followed from the second wave of alcohol policy liberalization were so remarkable in all three countries that the consequences were plainly obvious. Public opinion shifted back to more cautious tones about availability, state committees were set up to investigate the situation, and the growth in the number of monopoly shops and on-sale licences was frozen.

The policy theory adopted to respond to the situation was inspired by French alcohol policy, based on the work by the demographer Sully Ledermann. He had argued in the 1950s that the distribution of alcohol consumption is skewed and constant. Therefore, when the average consumption rate in a population increases, the number and consumption level of problem drinkers and the prevalence of drinking problems will increase even more. The objective of alcohol policy therefore should be to regulate the total consumption of a population, by means of taxation, opening hours and the network of outlets where alcoholic beverages are served or sold (Bruun et al. 1975).

Epidemiological research was conducted widely, comparing different kinds of populations and studying changes in consumption rates and distributions, usually with confirming results. Practical policy measures that followed included shorter business hours and tightened rules for serving and advertising alcohol, lower alcohol content of beer (Sweden), and high taxation of alcoholic beverages. The number of monopoly shops was stabilized.

From the Nordic countries the total consumption model spread to Canada, USA, UK and, incidentally, back to France where the alcohol and tobacco legislation of 1990 banned advertisements and introduced availability restrictions on the basis of this theory. In 1992 the European Regional Office of the World Health Organization accepted the First

Alcohol Action Plan, aiming at a 25 per cent reduction in the total consumption of alcohol in the region by the year 2000.

Bracketing out desire

The total consumption doctrine, as it came to be called, represented a radical change in the mode of restrictive approach in social control compared to the older pastoral regime. Alcohol use is, in this approach, considered a private matter and should be left to individuals – there is no preference for total abstinence, and the target is explicitly set at rates of consequences in the *population* rather than at drinking itself or individual problems. Among the consequences, health was prioritized, but again at the population level – this was often called the 'public health' approach. Alcohol is a public issue only insofar as the harmful consequences are concerned, and to deal with them the state should adopt methods that treat all citizens equally (Tigerstedt 1999). In this sense, even the backlash period in the 1970s that represents a non-liberal turn in availability policy with respect to the free market, was an instance of *political* liberalism: consumers were controlled only as members of the population, not as individuals, and only in the interest of the national political community, not in the interest of the naturally good life.

The equivalent in general welfare state research was called the 'resource theory'. Welfare was measured not in terms of outcomes, such as quality of work or housing, degree of education, family life or general satisfaction in life but in terms of the quantity and distribution of resources in the population. The desires were no longer classified as natural and artificial; in fact, for a long time there was complete silence on desires in social criticism as well as in the popular media. Desires were pushed underground, to the hidden sphere of private life; only the control of their consequences to the population was a public matter.

The new consumer society: emancipation of the self

The beginning of the 1980s marked the onset of a new, third kind of alcohol policy liberalism in all three Nordic monopoly countries. Newspapers started to run regular wine columns, popular associations for beer drinkers were founded, and the alcohol policy opinions began a new swing towards further market liberalization. The number of monopoly shops and bar licences started to increase again in the 1980s and restrictions on their business hours were eased. The alcohol retail monopoly in Finland adopted an active self-service policy, while Norway and Sweden proceeded more cautiously.

An important public debate took place in the early 1990s when these countries joined the EEA (Finland and Sweden also joined the EU in 1995), but the third liberal wave had commenced much earlier. The early 1980s marked a turn in public opinion concerning the state's role in regulating private consumption in a more general way. The change concerned especially public drinking places – restaurants, bars and pubs. For example, in Stockholm the number of on-licence outlets grew from about 400 in 1980 to 1,200 in 1990 (Abrahamsson 1999), and in Norway and Finland the number of public drinking places also grew rapidly.

Pleasure exposed

The third liberal wave differed from the preceding one in that, instead of references to the effects of policy measures, now the pleasure of drinking that had earlier been a strictly private matter became public. The debate on the population model had concerned only whether control was better than freedom in terms of the adverse consequences of drinking. Some had argued that control only makes alcohol more attractive as a 'forbidden fruit', whereas others attempted to show, often referring to research, that control works. How people would use the pleasures of drinking remained a private issue, just like the pleasures of sexuality. Until quite recently, sex education had also been discussed in terms of its effects on abortions and sexually transmitted diseases, not in terms of how important sexual satisfaction is to health and happiness.[4]

The whole experience of drinking, tasting, wine excursions and social-izing in drinking contexts is now the object of public discourse, and the desires that are satisfied by the uses of alcohol are placed on public display. 'Taste' is no longer an objective category assigned to the commodity; it is a subjective experience that requires both competence and ability – the competence referring to the many skills that make the appreciation possible, and the ability referring to the external circumstances that are necessary for the exercise of these skills.

The elite view from below

Public wine or whisky tastings, drink journalism and beer associations are new and significant phenomena because they introduce a perspective on alcohol policy that is quite different from the top-down civilizing liberalism of the 1950s and the radical egalitarian and expert-driven liberalism of the late 1960s and 1970s. They approach alcohol policy from the consumers' point of view, rather than from the perspective of moral authorities or experts representing the public good. The consumers' perspective is an elite point of view from below, arguing that we are now the civilized, competent and self-controlling sovereign citizens and consumers that the civilizing policy once set out to produce. The traditional external controls are, from that point of view, an insult imposed from above by bureaucrats, politicians and especially the temperance lobby, challenging this sovereignty and preventing its progress among those who still have to learn it.

Consumer emancipation

This way of arguing from a position below, while claiming the sovereignty of 'adulthood', has been common in alcohol-related editorials in journals as well as in interview studies (Sulkunen 1992). It produces a rhetoric of struggle for consumer emancipation. Liberal editorials on alcohol in Finnish dailies in the early 1990s were structured as narratives where the civilized consumers' rights are threatened by the elites, and the journal invites the readers to join the majority in completing the task of emancipation. The objective is to achieve the problem-free continental drinking culture with free availability of reasonably priced alcohol. The story is left pending, urging the readers for action, or at least for accepting the liberal opinion (Törrönen 2000).

In Sweden and Norway liberal arguments stress that the restricted availability has not worked and the people are demanding a change. Responsibility should be placed on the individual, and the state's role is to wake the consumers' own interest in protecting their health. In this view, regulating availability does not require a state monopoly as private ownership of the shops would have the same effect. However, controlling total consumption today is very difficult, and instead the emphasis should be placed on point abstinence (*punktnykterhet*) and lower alcohol content in beverages.

Management of the self

The obvious consequence of these claims has been support for private market interests, but from the point of view of governmental rationality, the neo-liberal ethos of the consumer society goes much deeper. It enlarges the territory of the managerial logic of the market to the whole spectrum of life, including not only the individuals' relationships to commodities, to the state and to others, but also to themselves. The neo-liberal consumers not only value free choice, they are also managers of themselves in two respects: first, they are managers of their satisfactions, which explains the prominence of the pleasures of drinking and sexuality, among the many other skills and competences of enjoyment that fill the media; second, they are managers of their aptitudes as competent and performing producer–consumers (Gordon 1991: 44). The 'public health' that was in the focus of the population-centred model of alcohol policy has now turned into an obligation to 'care for the self', which includes the psychological techniques of self-awareness and performance (Petersen and Lupton 1996).

In the alcohol issue the duality of self-management is particularly obvious. The management of satisfactions produces an enormous wealth of public discourse on the pleasures while the management of aptitudes produces an imperative of private self-control. The comments of one of the persons interviewed about their views of what constitutes the most serious drinking problems and what should be done about them are instructive. (The study was conducted among middle-class young adults in Finland in 1996.) One of those interviewed said: 'I think the cirrhosis is not even a problem, like lung cancer is not either', meaning that the real problem is not the consequences to health of excessive smoking or drinking. The real problem is the successful management of those pleasures (Sulkunen 1997).

Discussion

In the Nordic societies the state has had a strong role in promoting a good modern life throughout the twentieth century, and an alcohol control policy has been an exceptionally important part of this role. However, the governmental rationalities that have determined the logic of the alcohol–political reasoning have not been singularly Nordic. The civilizing policy and the policing of desires was, in fact, based on a relatively straightforward heritage from the Enlightenment, and parallel instances could be easily pointed out in sexual policies or education elsewhere. The population model since the 1960s has been a particular case of what, after Foucault, has been called 'biopolitics', and the neo-liberal elements in the contemporary alcohol policy discourses in the Nordic countries certainly are not unique when compared with other pleasures or other countries. The analysis in this chapter also overlooks the fact that there may be more divergencies, particularly concerning the neo-liberal consumer society, between the Nordic countries than between them and some other advanced societies, Finland being in this respect much more neo-liberal than Sweden or Norway.

From a comparative perspective, the important issue is the extent to which the shifts in governmental rationality described here translate into similar shifts in the other branches of the welfare state: income maintenance programmes and public services. This question is of special importance in the Nordic context because of the scale of the welfare programmes, but it is a key to understanding the morality and trajectories of welfare states anywhere.

Notes

1 Prohibition was a serious political option in all the temperance cultures that Levine (1992) analysed in Britain, the USA, Canada, Australia and New Zealand, and in the Nordic countries of Iceland, Norway, Sweden and Finland. Sweden never had a prohibition but instituted other forms of rigorous availability controls. The Norwegian prohibition (1916–1927) remained partial, excluding wine and beer (Fuglum 1995). In Switzerland, Austria and Germany

(partial) prohibitions were proposed but never gained wide political support (Eisenbach-Stangl 1991; Roberts 1984; Spode 1993).

2   The market-leading brewery Pripps was in fact 'nationalized' in 1974 by Olof Palme's government. However, the initiative came from the company itself, facing the uncertainty of the government's beer policy (Sulkunen 2000).

3   Gilles Lipovetsky (1992) has argued that modernity has been a deontic age that now is disintegrating. A diversity of obligations have structured the social order: obligations to God, to the Nation, to Progress, to Humanity, etc.

4   Until the early 1970s, sex counselling by Finnish medical doctors often took a normative stand on the kind of sex that is acceptable and who should be allowed to use contraceptives. The abortion law of 1970 quickly refocused the medical discourse on risks rather than pleasures (Warpenius, forthcoming).

References

Abrahamsson, M. (1999) *Alkoholkontroll i brytningstrid – ett kultursociologist perspektiv* (Alcohol control in transition – a cultural prespective), Stockholms Universitet.

Allardt, E. (1998) 'Det goda samhället. Välfärd, livsstil och medborgardygder' (The public good. Wefare, lifestyle and civil virtues), *Tidsskrift för Velfedsforskning*, 1, 3: 123–33.

Ambjörnsson, R. (1988) *Den skötsamme arbetaren. Idéer och ideal i ett norrländst sågverksamhälle 1880–1930* (The conscientious worker. Ideas and ideals in a northern sawmill community 1880–1930), Stockholm: Carlssons.

Anttila, A.-H. and Sulkunen, P. (2001) 'Alcohol policy in political parties' programmes', *Contemporary Drug Problems*, 28, 2.

Barrows, S. (1991) 'Parliaments of the people. The political culture of cafés in the early Third Republic', in S. Barrows and R. Room (eds) *Drinking Behaviour and Belief in Modern History*, Berkeley: University of California Press.

Bell, D. (1976) *The Cultural Contradictions of Capitalism*, New York: Basic Books.

Brennan, T. (1989) *Public Drinking and Popular Culture in Eighteenth Century Paris*, New Jersey: Princeton University Press.

Bruun, K. *et al.* (1975) *Alcohol Control Policy in Public Health Perspective*, Helsinki: Finnish Foundation for Alcohol Studies.

—— (1985) *Den svenska supen* (The Swedish drink), Stockholm: Prisma.

Campbell, C. (1987) *The Romantic Ethic and the Spirit of Modern Consumerism*, Cambridge: Basil Blackwell.

Dingle, A.E. (1980) *The Campaign for Prohibition in Victorian England. The United Kingdom Alliance 1872–1895*, London: Croom Helm.

Dorchester, D. (1884) *The Liquor Problem in All Ages*, New York: Phillips Hunt.

Eisenbach-Stangl, I. (1991) *Eine Gesellschaftsgeschichte des Alkohols. Produktion, Konsum und soziale Kontrolle alkoholischer Rausch- und Genussmittel in Österreich 1918–1984* (A social history of alcohol. Production, consumption and social control of alcoholic drinks in Austria 1918–1984), Frankfurt and New York: Campus Verlag.

Esping-Andersen, G. (1990) *The Three Worlds of Welfare Capitalism*, Cambridge: Polity Press.

Foucault, M. (1970) *The Order of Things: An Archaeology of the Human Sciences*, trans. A. Sheridan, London: Tavistock.

—— (1987) 'Politics and reason', in L.D. Kritzman (ed.) *Politics, Philosophy, Culture: Interviews and Other Writings*, New York: Routledge.

—— (1991) 'Governmentality', in G. Burchell, C. Gordon and P. Miller (eds) *The Foucault Effect*, Chicago: The University of Chicago Press.

Fuglum, P. (1995) *Brennevinsforbudet i Norge* (The Spirits Prohibition in Norway), Trondheim: Tapir Forlag.

Gellner, E. (1988) *Nations and Nationalism*, Oxford: Basil Blackwell.

Gordon, C. 'Governmental rationality: an introduction', in G. Burchell, C. Gordon and P. Miller (eds) *The Foucault Effect*, Chicago: The University of Chicago Press.

Gusfield, J. (1963) *Symbolic Crusade. Status Politics and the American Temperance Movement*, Westport, Connecticut: Greenwood Press.

Gutzke, D.W. (1989) *Protecting the Pub: Brewers and Publicans against Temperance*, Royal Historical Society, Studies in History, Suffolk: The Boydell Press.

Hamran, O. and Myrvang, C. (1988) *Fiin gammel vinmonopolet 75 år* (The fine old Norwegian alcohol monopoly 75 years), Oslo: Tano Aschehoug.

Harrison, B. (1971) *Drink and the Victorians. The Temperance Question in England 1815–1872* London: Faber.

Hauge, R. (1998) *Norsk alkohollovgivning gjennom 1000 år*, Oslo: Rusmiddeldirektoratet.

Heikkilä, M. *et al.* (1998) *Nordic Social Policy. Changing Welfare States*, London: Routledge.

Hirdman, Y. (1997) 'A social planning under rational control. Social engineering in Sweden in the 1930s and 1940s', in P. Kettunen and H. Eskola (eds) *Models, Modernity and the Myrdals*, Helsinki: Renvall Institute, University of Helsinki.

Hofstadter, R. (1955) *The Age of Reform*, New York: Vintage Books.

Holder, H., Kühlhorn, E., Nordlund, S., Österberg, E., Romelsjö, A. and Ugland, T. (1998) *European Integration and Nordic Alcohol Policies. Changes in Alcohol Control and Consequences in Finland, Norway and Sweden*, Aldershot: Ashgate.

Järvinen, M. (1991) 'Kontrollerade kontrollörer – kvinnor, män och alkohol' (Controlled controllers – women, men and alcohol), *Nordisk alkoholtidskrift*, 8: 143–52.

Johansson, L. (1992) *Brännvin, postillor och röda fanor* (Spirits, pulpits and red flag), Växjö: Högskolan i Växjö.

—— (2000) 'Sources of the Nordic solutions', in P. Sulkunen, Ch. Tigerstedt, C. Sutton and K. Warpenius (eds) *Broken Spirits. Power and Ideas in Nordic Alcohol Control*, Helsinki: NAD.

Lambert, W.R. (1983) *Drink and Sobriety in Victorian Wales 1820–1895*, Cardiff: University of Wales Press.

Levine, H. (1978) 'The discovery of addiction. Changing conceptions of habitual drunkenness in America', *Journal of Studies on Alcohol*, 39, 1: 143–74.

—— (1992) 'Temperance cultures: concern about alcohol problems in Nordic and English-speaking cultures', in M. Lader, G. Edwards and C. Drummond (eds) *The Nature of Alcohol and Drug Related Problems*, New York: Oxford University Press.

Lipovetsky, G. (1992) *Le crépuscule du devoir* (The dusk of obligation), Paris: Gallimard.

Magnusson, L. (1985) 'Orsaker till det förindustriella drickandet. Supandet i hautverkets Eskilstuna' (Causes of pre-industrial drinking), *Alkoholpolitik*, 23, 1: 23–9.

Mäkelä, K. (1976) *Alkoholipoliittisen mielipideilmaston vaihtelut Suomessa 1960-ja 70-luvulla* (Alcohol policy opinions in Finland in the 1960s and 1970s), Alkoholipoliittisen tutkimuslaitoksen tutkimusseloste (Reports of the Social Research Institute of Alcohol Studies No. 98, Helsinki).

Mills, C.W. (1958) *The Sociological Imagination*, Glencoe: Free Press.

Myrdal, A. and Myrdal, G. (1935) *Kris i befolkningsfrågan* (The crisis in the population question), Stockholm: Albert Bonniers Förlag.

Nycander, S. (1996) *Svenskarna och spriten. Alkoholpolitik 1855–1995* (Alcohol and the Swedes. Alcohol policy 1855–1995), Stockholm: Sober.

Paton, D.N. (1977) *Drink and the Temperance Movement in nineteenth century Scotland*, unpublished PhD thesis, University of Edinburgh.

Peltonen, M. (1991) 'Kieli vai kulttuuri? Väittely suomalaisesta viinapäästä keväällä 1948' (Language or culture. The debate on the Finnish drinking patterns in 1948), *Alkoholipolitiikka*, 56: 8–25.

Petersen, A. and Lupton, D. (1996) *The New Public Health. Health and Self in the Age of Risk*, London: Sage.

Ragnarsson, L. (1993) *Från motbok till snabbköp* (From rationing to self-service), Stockholm: Systembolaget.

Raphael, D.D. and Macfie, A.L. (1984) 'Introduction', in A. Smith (ed.) *The Theory of Moral Sentiments*, Indianapolis: Liberty Fund.

Roberts, J. (1984) *Drink, Temperance and the Working Class in 19th Century Germany*, London: Allen & Unwin.

Rose, K.D. (1997) *American Women and the Repeal of Prohibition*, New York: New York University Press.

Rose, N. (1999) *Powers of Freedom: Reframing Political Thought*, Cambridge: Cambridge University Press.

Rosenzweig, R. (1983) *Eight Hours for What We Will. Workers and Leisure in an Industrial City 1870–1920*, Cambridge: Cambridge University Press.

Roszak, Th. (1968) *The Making of a Counter-Culture*, Berkeley: University of California Press.

Shiman, L.L. (1988) *Crusade Against Drink in Victorian England*, London: Macmillan.

Slagstad, R (1998) *De nasjonale strateger* (The national strategists), Oslo: Pax Forlag.

Smith, A. (1984) *The Theory of Moral Sentiments*, Indianapolis: Liberty Fund.

Smout, T.C. (1986) *A Century of the Scottish People*, London: Fontana Press.

Spode, H. (1993). *Die Macht der Trunkenheit. Kultur- und Sozialgeschichte des Alkohols in Deutschland* (The power of drunkenness. Cultural and social history of alcohol in Germany), Opladen: Ledke & Budrich.

Stenius, K. (1999) *Privat och offentligt i svensk alkoholistvård*, Lund: Arkiv.

Sulkunen, I. (1986) *Raittus kansalaisuskontona. Raittiusliikkeen järjestäytyminen 1870-luvulta suurlakon jälkeisiin vuosiin* (Temperance as a civil religion. The organisation of temperance movement between 1870 and the General Strike of 1906), Helsinki: Societas Historica Finlandiae.

Sulkunen, P. (1992) *The European New Middle Class*, Ashgate: Aldershot.

—— (1997) 'Logics of prevention: mundane speech and expert discourse on alcohol policy', in P. Sulkunen, J. Holmwood, H. Radner and G. Schulze, (eds) *Constructing the New Consumer Society*, London: Macmillan.

—— (2000) 'The Liberal arguments', in P. Sulkunen, Ch. Tigerstedt, C. Sutton and K. Warpenius (eds) *Broken Spirits. Power and Ideas in Nordic Alcohol Control*, Helsinki: NAD.

Sulkunen, P., Tigerstedt, Ch., Sutton, C. and Warpenius, K. (eds) (2000) *Broken Spirits. Power and Ideas in Nordic Alcohol Control*, Helsinki: NAD.

Sulkunen, P. and Warpenius, K. (2001) 'Controlling the self and the other. Temperance movements and the duality of modern individuality', *Critical Public Health*, 1.

Tigerstedt, C. (1999) 'Alcohol policy, public health and Kettil Bruun', *Contemporary Drug Problems*, 26, 2: 209–35.

Timberlake, J.H. (1963) *Prohibition and the Progressive Movement, 1900–1920*, Cambridge, Mass.: Harvard University Press.

Törrönen, J. (2000) 'The passionate text: the pending narrative as a macrostructure of persuasion', *Social Semiotics*, 10, 1.

Valverde, M. (1998) *Diseases of the Will: Alcohol and the Dilemmas of Freedom*, Cambridge: Cambridge University Press.

Warpenius, K. (forthcoming) 'From pleasure to risk. Alcohol policy and sex education in Finland 1965–1975', *Acta Sociologica*.

Weber, M. (1970) *The Protestant Ethic and the Spirit of Capitalism*, trans. T. Parsons, London: Routledge & Kegan Paul.

Chapter 5

Mental health consumers or citizens with mental health problems?

Mike Hazelton and Michael Clinton

In 1997 and 1998 the authors participated in a series of Australian Commonwealth Government-funded workshops designed to set future directions for the education and training of the mental health professions in Australia (Deakin Human Services Australia 1999). Five mental health professions – psychiatry, psychology, mental heath nursing, social work and occupational therapy – were equally represented in each of the three main workshops. What made the project unique, at least in the experience of the authors, was the high level of direct participation by persons who were (a) the direct users of mental health services (referred to in the workshops as 'consumers') or (b) provided lay support to the users of mental health services (referred to in the workshops as 'carers'). However, despite this high level of participation by consumers and carers it is doubtful that the recommendations of the project, as specified in the Final Report (Deakin Human Services Australia 1999), have had, or will have, any significant impact in influencing the direction of education and training for the mental health professions in Australia. The chapter examines some of the reasons for this apparent lack of impact. Recent Australian mental health policy frames the users of mental health services as 'consumers' exercising 'choice', as if mental health services were 'products' in a kind of health care market place, and this health consumer model operated implicitly and explicitly as the business of the workshops unfolded. It will be argued, however, that the apparent lack of impact of the project can be understood in relation to concerns regarding the applicability of health consumerism to mental health care.

The chapter begins by discussing the purpose and outcomes of the Education and Training Partnerships in Mental Health Workshops (Deakin Human Services Australia 1999). This is followed by a discussion of the idea of mental health consumerism in current mental health policy. While the recent changes in mental health policy – including the introduction of health consumerism – represent a significant policy change, public and professional support for the changes should not be assumed. Indeed, there is some evidence that policy changes designed to liberalize and rationalize mental health services have contributed to rising concerns regarding the risks posed by mentally ill persons living in the community. These issues surrounding what has been referred to as the post-liberal turn in mental health policy and practice are considered in later sections of the chapter. The chapter concludes with a discussion of prospects for realizing the citizenship and human rights project at the heart of recent mental health policy changes in Australia.

The Education and Training Partnerships Project

While consumer involvement in all aspects of service planning, delivery and evaluation has been identified as a priority in the National Mental Health Strategy (Australian Health Ministers 1992a), policy-makers have expressed concern that initiatives designed to achieve this outcome are not being taken up in the mental health workforce. Much greater emphasis should be given to increasing the responsiveness of the workforce to consumer concerns, outlooks and needs. As the (then) Commonwealth Director of Mental Health asserted, mental health professionals should accept:

> that people with [severe mental illness] have 'expert' knowledge, they have individual needs and expectations. Furthermore, consumers and their carers can contribute greatly to the recovery and management of mental illness as well as to the quality of the care delivered by the professional workforce ... Fostering a culture which values the opinions of consumers and carers must be the overarching goal of continued reform in this area.
>
> (cited in Deakin Human Services Australia 1999: i)

The Education and Training Partnerships Project (hereafter referred to as the Partnerships Project) emerged out of the perceived failure of an earlier project addressing workforce development and education and training issues in the Australian mental health workforce (KMPG Consulting 1994). The earlier report had been widely criticized for 'ignoring the roles of universities and professional associations, the experiences and views of consumers and carers and the different roles of the disciplines' (Deakin Human Services Australia 1999: 4). The Partnerships Project was thus envisaged as a kind of rescue mission which would bring together key representatives of each of the main mental health disciplines, including the university sector, the professional colleges and organizations, government officials and policy-makers and consumers and carers. The objectives of the Partnerships Project were (a) to facilitate improvements in education and training in the five major disciplines practising in the mental health field; (b) to meet the needs of consumers and carers exposed to severe mental illness; and (c) to outline the structural and policy 'drivers' for progress in this area (Deakin Human Services Australia 1999: 4).

The project unfolded as a series of consultative workshops, which sought consensus regarding possible options for increasing consumer and carer participation in all levels of education and training in each of the five participating mental health disciplines. Three main workshops were conducted comprising eight representatives from each professional discipline, eight consumers and eight carers. Each disciplinary group (except psychiatry) also held an additional mini-workshop focusing on discipline-specific issues.

While much time was taken up in discussing professional rivalries and relationships between service providers and service users, a (fragile) consensus was achieved regarding the principles that should guide future education and training for the mental health professions: the relationships between consumers and service providers and carers and service providers, should be the primary focus of practice and research in mental health. Consumers and carers are therefore major players in the education, training and development of the mental health workforce. Following on from this broad statement of principle, future determinations of the effectiveness of education and training for the mental health disciplines must stress that mental health professionals: need to learn about and value the lived experience of consumers and carers; and should recognize and value the healing potential in the relationships between consumers and service providers and carers and service providers (Deakin Human Services Australia 1999: 5).

Each of the mental health discipline groups undoubtedly experienced these principles as challenging. While each group eventually supported the principles (at least within the context of the workshops), it was not clear how this would translate into actual proposals for reviewing current or future curricula. At the time of writing, more than two years after the release of the Final Report (Deakin Human Services Australia 1999), there is little evidence of the Partnerships Project having influenced education and training in any of the mental health professions. While the idea of consumer participation in professional education and training and clinical service provision might appear to have gained political and managerial support, this has not necessarily carried over into the everyday world of university educators and mental health personnel.

There are thus good reasons for questioning whether the politics of psychiatric care are likely to be supportive of the kind of enabling programme envisaged in the Partnerships Project. On the one hand, concerns have been raised regarding whether the field of mental health care can be, or should be, transformed into a kind of health enterprise, complete with 'mental health consumers' and 'health service providers'. On the other hand, it is doubtful that mental heath personnel will turn away from their traditional roles as psychiatric experts and embrace a power-sharing arrangement involving those for whom they provide clinical services. These issues, which were very much at the heart of Partnerships Project, are taken up in greater detail in the following sections.

Mental health policy and health consumerism

The concerns addressed in the Partnerships Project should be seen as part of an international trend in mental health policy reform. In recent decades mental health systems in many countries have been transformed as governments have implemented policies through which to coordinate and direct the development of services. While such policies reflect local requirements, they also exhibit a number of similar concerns, including: sensitivity to human rights issues; commitment to service development and continuous quality improvement; insistence on service accountability; pursuit of cost effectiveness, and redeveloping mental health services to become part of mainstream health services.

Following these international trends, the policy focus in Australia's *National Mental Health Strategy* (Australian Health Ministers 1992a) has been on shifting psychiatric services into the general health sector; forging links between psychiatric services, general health services, and other non-health services such as housing and social security; improving continuity of care across the range of providers of mental health care and safeguarding and enhancing the rights of people who are mentally ill. A second phase of the Strategy that commenced in 1998 reconfirmed these policy priorities, but gave greater emphasis to a population health perspective, continuous quality improvement and the need to improve health professionals' attitudes towards the mentally ill (Commonwealth Department of Health and Aged Care 2000).

The mental health policy framework that emerged in the 1990s identified consumers' needs and rights as a priority. The development of strategies for consumer representation, protection against discrimination and adoption of safeguards and rights, such as those contained in the United Nations Principles for the Protection of Persons with Mental Illness (United Nations General Assembly 1992), were seen as crucial. As was noted in the *Mental Health Statement of Rights and Responsibilities* (Australian Health Ministers 1991: viii), people with severe mental illness have traditionally 'had limited say, and in some cases, little choice about the nature and form of services they received. These decisions ... generally rested with health and welfare professionals and service administrators.' Ensuring equity, access and social justice for people who use mental health services now became an important governmental concern: '[it] is essential to ensure that their needs for care, protection and rights to treatment and rehabilitation are satisfied. The diagnosis of mental health problems or mental disorder is not an excuse for inappropriately limiting their rights' (Australian Health Ministers 1991: ix). Accordingly, mentally ill people must be given the 'opportunity to live, work and participate in the community to the full extent of their capabilities without discrimination' (Australian Health Ministers 1992a: 16).

By bringing together a range of interconnected themes involving social justice, stigma, discrimination, human rights and the vulnerability of, and need to protect the mentally ill, the policy discourse of the *National Mental Health Strategy* highlighted the role of government as a protector of rights. There is, however, an important contradiction here. On the one hand, governments are seeking to work 'in partnership with consumers, carers, and service providers, to ensure that people with a mental illness ... enjoy the same rights, choices, and opportunities as other Australians' (Australian Government 1994: iii). On the other hand, 'government accepts ... that people affected by mental illness are among the most vulnerable and disadvantaged in our community' (Australian Government 1994: 10). Two constructions of the mentally ill emerge from this mental health policy discourse. One, a 'consumer' of services, enjoys 'the [same] rights, choices, and opportunities' as other citizens. The other, constituted as powerless, is vulnerable to discrimination and various rights infringements. One, having wishes, wants and desires, will actively pursue these. The other, being vulnerable and having needs, requires protection.

The mental health policy framework also depicts mental illness as being both a personal problem and an important issue for the community (Australian Health Ministers 1991). Good mental health is seen as a kind of commodity form; it is both a personal resource and an important community and national asset: '[the] cost of mental disorder is significant in economic and social terms for individuals, their families and the community' (Australian Health Ministers 1992b: 4). Supporting the community in improving the mental health of its members is thus seen as a major investment in all aspects of community life (Australian Health Ministers 1991: vii). Not only was the importance of safeguarding the citizenship and human rights of persons with mental illness fully acknowledged within the Partnerships Project, it was seen as being central to the aims of the workshops:

> people with mental illness are primarily citizens, with full citizenship and social rights ... Acceptance of this tenet means that the disciplines working in mental health are now obliged to meet not only the professionally defined needs of a person with mental illness but also to recognize inherent civil, political and social rights.
>
> (Deakin Human Services Australia 1999: 12)

The extension of human rights and citizenship rights to the mentally ill has thus become a central feature of recent mental health policy in countries such as Australia. However, we will argue that the preferred form of 'citizenship' envisaged in the reforms reflects the 'enterprisation' of public benefits and services that has been introduced throughout the public sector during the last decade or more, and that this has serious implications for the social justice aims of the policy. What are the implications of reconstituting the mentally ill as 'consumers', active citizens participating in the kind of health enterprise culture envisaged in recent health policy?

Mental health consumers?

As mentioned above, recent Australian mental health policy constructs the person with mental problems and disorders as a consumer of services, an active individual who enjoys the same citizenship rights, responsibilities and challenges as any other citizen. At the same time, however, this same subject is also represented as being powerless, vulnerable and in need of protection. Some commentators have noted an affinity between the structural form 'health consumer' found in health policy, and that of the consumer found in marketing discourse (Grace 1991). The underlying concepts and assumptions concerning relations between 'consumers' and 'providers' have been seen to parallel the broad logic of capitalist market relations (Grace 1991; Pilgrim and Rogers 1993: 165–71), thus reflecting the wide-ranging process of commodifying welfare services that has long been underway throughout liberal-democratic industrialized states (Pilgrim and Rogers 1993: 165, citing Offe 1984). For Grace (1991: 334), this type of reconceptualization neutralizes possibilities for resistance, by effecting a (discursive) shift from the terrain of political challenge to that of the market relation. On this new terrain the (collective) 'demands' of mental health advocates and activists become the (individual) 'needs' of mental health 'consumers'. Drawing on Turner's (1990) typology of citizenship, these developments can be understood as the displacement of forms of citizenship developed from below, with those structured from above.

While mental health policy is overtly geared towards enhancing public participation in (mental) health, the officially preferred option for achieving this turns out to be heavily bureaucratically structured, and therefore seems likely to contribute to the further entrenchment of dominant interests and governmental concerns. This type of 'structured community participation in health' constructs the consultative process in ways that reduce 'consumer involvement ... to a relatively passive process that does not, of itself, enable the imbalances of power to be challenged' (Willis 1995: 213). Moreover, Willis (1995: 214) suggests that bureaucratically structured forms of community participation can also work towards neutralizing competing (political) interests by co-optation. While dissatisfaction with mental health services has been expressed through the emergence of the mental health movements, both locally and internationally (Rogers et al. 1993), these are constantly at risk of political neutralization through being drawn into the corporate structures of the state health sector.

It has been argued that while recent policy developments in countries such as Australia and the United Kingdom acknowledge the rights of the mentally ill, the operational commitment to the idea of user participation and consultation remains very limited (Rogers *et al.* 1993). Thus, while recent mental health policy seems to be consumer focused, 'health authorities ... need only incorporate a consumer perspective when, and if it is expedient' (Rogers *et al.* 1993: 2). The implication here, of course, is that attempts by state officials and health professionals to (apparently) facilitate the taking of control by the people, may turn out to be pseudo-participation, heavily structured by those in positions of state or professional authority (Dwyer 1989; Willis 1995). Thus, when managers and clinical personnel claim to be responding to the needs of the mentally ill, and wider public concerns over the provision of mental health care, the institutional positioning of these officials is likely to result in the further entrenching of official interests (Willis 1995).

A key aspect of recent health reforms in countries such as Australia, New Zealand and the United Kingdom has been the introduction of an enterprise culture into the provision of health care (Grace 1991; Davis 1992; Fougere 1992; Hicks 1995). The expectation here 'is that by forcing providers to compete for purchasers' business, a more efficient provision of health care will result, since, in theory, purchasers will only offer contracts to those institutions that operate in an efficient manner' (Shackley and Ryan 1994: 519). While the efficiency imperative has often dominated discussions surrounding health reforms both locally and internationally (Davis 1992), the success of market-styled reforms depends heavily on whether health service users will, or can, act as 'good consumers', that they will 'adequately assimilate information on the costs and the quality of health care, and on the basis of such information ... make health choices' (Shackley and Ryan 1994: 518).

As Petersen *et al.* point out in Chapter 7, the use of a consumer model in health care raises important questions, and this is especially so in respect of mental health services. While in their chapter Petersen *et al.* are especially concerned with issues of health consumerism, stigma and cultural difference, it should also be noted that, for many persons experiencing mental illness, engagement with mental health services is anything but a matter of choice. Unlike most other categories of health service user, those receiving mental health care are constantly at risk of having legally mandated restrictions placed on their personal liberty (and other civil rights) (Centre for Health Law, Ethics and Policy 1994). In such circumstances it can hardly be said that 'mental health consumers' are exercising 'choice'; that is, unless attempts to abscond from 'care' are interpreted in this light!

For many persons designated as mentally ill, the range of possible life experiences are simply incongruent with the ideas implicit within the notion of a 'health consumer'; these might include non-treatment, destitution and poverty, at one end of the scale, to involuntary hospitalization, forced treatment and being subjected to legal orders, at the other end. For many, the developments associated with health consumerism – patient's charter of rights, advocacy, complaints processes, or more liberal mental health legislation – have not secured the power to choose. As two of the consumer participants in the Partnerships Project workshops indicated, '[mental health service] users have not become genuine consumers with purchasing power. Purchasing is done in our name. Our needs are represented for us ...' (Deakin Human Services Australia 1999: 23). Moreover, those who use mental health services often seem reluctant to describe themselves as consumers, preferring other terms such as 'service users', 'recipients' or 'survivors' (Campbell 1999: 17). Indeed, for a number of the consumer participants in the Partnerships Project, 'survivor' was the only service user identity grounded in the experience of those on the receiving end of psychiatric care (Deakin Human Services Australia 1999: 22). Campbell (1999: 18) has neatly summarized the problems associated with applying a health consumer model to mental health care:

> Unlike consumers in other markets, [the mentally ill] do not have the right to choose or withhold choice, to enter or exit the market. Focusing on the lives of people with a mental illness diagnosis as if they were pre-eminently consumers of care carries a real danger of totally missing the essential nature of their experience. A journey through a shopping mall and a journey through mental health services are simply worlds apart.

Power relations in mental health care

While the Partnerships Project was concerned with how the education and training of professionals working in the mental health field might be redeveloped to better meet the needs of those under psychiatric care, consumer and carer participants in the workshops stressed the extent to which the human rights aspects of mental health policy had so far had 'little impact at the level of everyday relations between providers and consumers' (Deakin Human Services Australia 1999: 36). From the discussions of the workshops it was clear that despite the introduction of apparently liberalizing reforms to mental health services throughout the last decade, many users of mental health services continue to experience mental health care as oppressive. At the same time, most of the professional participants at one stage or another admitted to feeling that the purpose of the workshops posed a threat to their professional power and traditional models of working (Deakin Human Services Australia 1999: 40). The power relations underpinning psychiatric care thus emerged time and again as issues throughout the workshops.

The era of the asylums is still within the living memory of many persons currently working in and receiving care from psychiatric services and, as

Cawte (1998: 16) has recently noted, the asylum system was one in which psychiatric professionals were both therapists and jailors. As the architects of the Partnerships Project acknowledged, the recent policy changes raise difficult questions regarding the relationship between mental health personnel and those under their care: '[The] groups with the most adverse attitudes to those with mental illness are ... their treating staff, those who "gatekeep" the facilities and services dealing with mental illness' (Deakin Human Services Australia 1999: 11). There is thus good reason to question the extent to which the new policy directions have trickled down to influence the mindsets and practices of personnel. Psychiatric personnel have traditionally worked with a notion of the mentally ill as vulnerable individuals requiring management and protection, with the consequence that:

> Professional preoccupations with the difficulties, problems and 'weaknesses' of consumers [have] rendered them passive recipients of services controlled by professionals who decided what [is] 'best'. The consequence for consumers has been that most community-based provision has replicated the all-too-familiar relationships of institutional life.
>
> (Davis 1988: 35, cited in Barham 1992: 64)

It has often been noted that the maintenance of social and psychological 'distance' between professionals and those receiving their services has been a defining feature of professional dominance (Deakin Human Services Australia 1999: 11). Indeed, for mental health personnel it is all too easy to disregard the opinions of the mentally ill as irrational, invalid, or even biased towards professional opinions (Pridmore 1990). Ultimately, however, the most effective foil against challenges to the authority of psychiatric expertise has been to invoke the (ideological) image of medical-scientific legitimacy; the expectation being that:

> [some one] in a lab ... will find a receptor that when properly stimulated clears thought disorders and stops auditory hallucinations, or they'll find a virus ... It's that solution that can solve the public policy problems.
>
> (Appelbaum, cited in Issac and Armat 1990: 345)

In general terms, psychiatric personnel have a somewhat unstable, even contrary relationship with the mentally ill. 'Even the way mental health workers designate those they treat and support shifts constantly: "patient", "client", "consumer", "service user". They have no stable identity vis-à-vis the system' (Coffey 1994: 34). Moreover, as the consumer participants in the Partnerships Project workshops noted, the experiences of the users of mental health services are also often 'interpreted as part of the "illness" for which [they] are being treated' (Deakin Human Services Australia 1999: 21). At the same time, however, the liberalization of ward policies and practices designed to promote patients' freedom of movement and expression, and the use of minimal sedation, can create more work and increased risks for staff. Indeed, security and risk management have become important issues for many mental health personnel, especially nurses, involved in the day-to-day care and control of the mentally ill (Hazelton 1999; Clinton and Hazelton 2000a; 2000b). The active promotion of patients' rights and the introduction of formal complaints procedures within mental health administrative procedures can also be experienced by staff as casting doubts on their professional integrity (Coffey 1994: 34).

It seems likely that the policy-driven pressures and tensions running through mental health services have also amplified the intensely political nature of psychiatric work. While at the broadest level, medical–psychiatric thought and practice continues to structure 'how things should be done' in mental health services, as with other health services, this is constantly open to challenge, resistance and modification (Turner 1987: 221–3; Wicks 1995). Non-medical personnel have at their disposal a range of tactics and strategies for holding medical authority in check, including forging strategic alliances with other non-medical occupations; the gradual modification over time of medical treatment orders; the selective and/or partial implementation of medical orders and even direct confrontation in which medically preferred management approaches are openly challenged by non-medical personnel. There is no doubt that patients get caught up in and are marginalized, or even 'demonized' within these intra-occupational struggles, especially when these involve disputes over the management of patients considered 'difficult' and/or 'dangerous' (Hazelton 1999). The likelihood of conflict between the mental health professions seems even greater in a period marked by upheavals and wide-ranging reorganization:

> In the past few decades ... mental health practitioners and managers have been expected to: accommodate the independent sector; disentangle purchasers from providers, and health care from social care; introduce care plans for patients discharged from hospital; offer non-custodial care and treatment to mentally disordered offenders; reduce morbidity and suicide rates; give priority to people placed on supervision registers; implement new mental health legislation; assess the risk of violence and homicide; provide 'seamless' care or a 'continuum' of care; respond to the implications of the patient's charter ... .
>
> (Morrall 2000: 19–20)

The emergence of post-liberal mental health policies, laws and practices

If the mental policy directions of the last few decades can be thought of as liberalizing the mental health field, there is evidence that we are already entering a post-liberal stage characterized by the identification, surveillance and exclusion of certain dangerous populations. Control measures may be considered 'post-liberal' if they are radically authoritarian, but operate within a democratic framework (Morrall and Hazelton 2000; Morrall 2000). Post-liberalism can therefore be understood as the incorporation of laws, policies and practices aimed at socially excluding demonized groups (i.e. those considered to pose a threat to the public order, especially where there is an actual or potential threat of violence). Examples of post-liberal laws and policies recently introduced in the United Kingdom include mandatory life-sentences for repeat serious violent or sexual offenders, police registers for sex offenders, and anti-social behaviour orders targeting juvenile offenders (Morrall 2000). These developments have also extended into the mental health field in the United Kingdom, in the form of supervision registers for severely mentally ill people living in the community and the (proposed) compulsory detention of people with personality disorder without trial and without a crime having been committed (Morrall 2000).

While the impact of post-liberalism has so far been limited in Australia's criminal justice system – for instance, in the 'three strikes and you're out' mandatory sentencing policy of the Northern Territory – there is some evidence of the trend influencing developments in mental health care. In one of the ironies of the mental health policy directions taken in Australia throughout the 1990s, the emergence of human rights concerns in psychiatric care coincided with the upgrading of security measures in many mental health facilities. Closed circuit television monitoring, security fences, the building of 'high dependency' units (i.e. seclusion units) and the routine use of duress alarms by staff all became commonplace throughout mental health services. Private sector security guards have been employed by some hospitals and it is not unusual for these personnel to be called to 'assist' in managing disturbed patients in mental health clinical areas (Hazelton 1999). So far the development of this security and surveillance infrastructure within mental health services in Australia has not attracted the attention of mental health policy-makers.

Mental health consumers or citizens with mental health problems?

The main purpose of the Partnerships Project was to facilitate improvements in the education and training of the mental health professions to better meet the needs of those who use mental health services. To this end, the project was concerned with exploring how consumers might be included as key stakeholders in the development and delivery of education and training curricula for the mental health professions. However, this chapter has raised questions regarding the prospects for the mentally ill engaging with mental health personnel on anything like equal terms within the kind of 'consumer driven' enterprise culture envisaged in recent mental health policy, whether this be in the realm of clinical service delivery or in education and training.

While enabling projects such as the Partnerships Project officially acknowledge that 'severe mental illness need no longer be a barrier to ordinary human recognition and the entitlements of citizenship' (Barham 1992: 100), it is not clear that the life circumstances of mentally ill persons are changing for the better. Indeed, it has been argued that the recent policy changes may have placed the mentally ill in a citizenship 'no man's land', conferring a kind of approximate or 'as if' citizenship. Barham (1992: 101, citing Lewis *et al.* 1989: 173–4) is thinking of this type of marginal citizenship when he suggests that despite the progressive policy directions of recent decades the mentally ill largely remain a mystery:

> We do not know them, because they are neither outside society in the world of exclusion, nor are they full citizens – individuals who are like the rest of us. Being neither other nor self, they are a new kind of social construction.

As Campbell (1999: 24) points out, the extent to which citizenship may be available to mentally ill people 'depends not only on the degree of shelter, support and occupational opportunity provided by community care services but on the attitudes that inspire those facilities and inform public opinion'. He goes on to suggest that the limits of public tolerance for mentally ill people living in the community may already have been reached: 'It is possible that enthusiasm for the rights and the contribution of mental patients has already passed its peak' (Campbell 1999: 24). Moreover, traditional assumptions regarding the association between insanity and criminality – madness and badness – continue to find expression in occasional moral panics regarding the risks posed by the unsupervised mentally ill. Morrall (2000) has recently explored the moral panic surrounding homicides perpetrated by mentally ill offenders in the United Kingdom and how this has influenced the trend towards the development of the kinds of post-liberal mental health policies and legislation discussed in the preceding section.

Finally, it is important to question how mental health personnel might be managing the new policy directions. Far from simply implementing policy dictates handed down from above, mental health personnel seem likely to engage in a kind of enacted policy, actively reshaping, modifying, ignoring and undermining policy initiatives (Hazelton 1999). The response of personnel to apparently liberalizing reforms may well be in the direction of being more guarded and secretive about their practices. There was some evidence of this in the Partnerships Project, with some professional participants, especially the psychiatrists, appearing less willing than others to engage in workshop activities (Deakin Human Services Australia 1999: 47).

There is also evidence of a post-liberal turn in mental health services in countries such as the United Kingdom and Australia. A kind of policy paradox in which the working out of apparently liberalizing policy initiatives designed to turn mental health services into enterprise cultures has coincided with the emergence of what might be thought of as a 'new institutionalism' (Morrall and Hazelton 2000) – complete with new forms of surveillance, security practices and social exclusions. It may well be that the more liberal policy environment that made initiatives such as the Partnerships Project possible has already passed. It remains to be seen whether the mentally ill will benefit by being made to transact 'business' with their care-givers within a system of health care enterprise.

References

Australian Government (1994) *Working Together. Mental Health Federal Budget Initiatives 1994–95*, Canberra: Australian Government Publishing Service.
Australian Health Ministers (1991) *Mental Health Statement of Rights and Responsibilities*, Canberra: Australian Government Publishing Service.
—— (1992a) *National Mental Health Policy*, Canberra: Australian Government Publishing Service.
—— (1992b) *National Mental Health Plan*, Canberra: Australian Government Publishing Service.
Barham, P. (1992) *Closing the Asylum. The Mental Patient in Modern Society*, London: Penguin Books.
Campbell, P. (1999) 'The consumer of mental health care', in R. Newell and K. Gourney (eds) *Mental Health Nursing. An Evidence-Based Approach*, Edinburgh: Churchill Livingstone, pp. 11–26.
Cawte, J. (1998) *The Last of the Lunatics*, Melbourne: Melbourne University Press.
Centre for Health Law, Ethics and Policy (1994) *Model Mental Health Legislation. A Discussion Paper*, Centre for Health Law, Ethics and Policy: The University of Newcastle, Australia.
Clinton, M. and Hazelton, M. (2000a) 'Scoping the Australian mental health nursing workforce', *Australian and New Zealand Journal of Mental Health Nursing*, 9, 2: 56–64.
—— (2000b) 'Scoping practice issues in the Australian mental health nursing workforce', *Australian and New Zealand Journal of Mental Health Nursing*, 9, 3: 100–9.
Coffey, G. (1994) 'Madness and postmodern civilization', *Arena*, April–May: 32–7.
Commonwealth Department of Health and Aged Care (2000) *National Mental Health Report 2000: Sixth Annual Report. Changes in Australia's Mental Health Services under the First National Mental Health Plan of the National Mental Health Strategy 1993–1998*, Canberra: Australian Government Publishing Service.
Davis, A. (1992) 'Economising health', in S. Rees, G. Rodley and F. Stillwell (eds) *Beyond the Market. Alternatives to Economic Rationalism*, Leichhardt: Pluto Press.
Deakin Human Services Australia (1999) *Learning Together: Education and Training Partnerships in Mental Health Service*. Final report, prepared by Deakin Human

Services Australia with funding from the Commonwealth Department of Health and Aged Care under the National Mental Health Strategy. Canberra: Australian Government Printing Service.

Dwyer, J. (1989) The politics of community participation', *Community Health Studies*, 13, 1: 59–65.

Fougere, G. (1992) *The State and Health Care Reform*, unpublished paper presented as part of the Winter Lecture Series, The University of Auckland, New Zealand, 15 July 1992.

Grace, V.M. (1991) 'The marketing of empowerment and the construction of the health consumer: a critique of health promotion', *International Journal of Health Sciences*, 21, 2: 329–43.

Hazelton, M. (1999) 'Psychiatric personnel, risk management and the new institutionalism', *Nursing Inquiry*, 6: 224–30.

Hicks, N. (1995) 'Economism, managerialism and health care', *Annual Review of Social Science*, 5: 39–60.

Isaac, R.J. and Armat, V.C. (1990) *Madness in the Streets: How Psychiatry and the Law Abandoned the Mentally Ill*, New York: The Free Press.

KMPG Consulting (1994) *National Mental Health Workforce Education and Training Consultancy, Report*, unpublished Report, KMPG Consulting, Melbourne.

Morrall, P.A. (2000) *Madness and Murder*, London: Whurr.

Morrall, P.A. and Hazelton, M. (2000) 'Architecture signifying social control: the restoration of asylumdom in mental health care?', *Australian and New Zealand Journal of Mental Health Nursing*, 9, 2: 89–96.

Offe, C. (1984) *Contradictions of the Welfare State*, London: Hutchinson.

Pilgrim, D. and Rogers, A. (1993) *A Sociology of Mental Health and Illness*, Buckingham: Open University Press.

Pridmore, S. (1990) 'Mental health in the 1990s', *Mental Health in Australia*, 3, 1: 38–40.

Rogers, A., Pilgrim, D. and Lacey, R. (1993) *Experiencing Psychiatry: Users' Views of Services*, London: Macmillan.

Shackley, P. and Ryan, M. (1994) 'What is the role of the consumer in health care?', *Journal of Social Policy*, 23, 4: 517–41.

Turner, B.S. (1987) *Medical Power and Social Knowledge*, London: Sage.

—— (1990) 'Outline of a theory of citizenship', *Sociology*, 24, 2: 189–217.

United Nations General Assembly (1992) *Principles for the Protection of Persons with Mental Illness and for the Improvement of Mental Health Care*, New York: United Nations.

Wicks, D. (1995) 'Nurses, doctors and discourses of healing', *Australian and New Zealand Journal of Sociology*, 31, 2: 122–39.

Willis, K. (1995) 'Imposed structures and contested meanings: policies and politics of public participation', *Australian Journal of Social Issues*, 30: 211–27.

Part II

Consumerism in practice
Manifestations and experiences

Chapter 6

Consumerism in the hospital context

Saras Henderson

Introduction

Contemporary thinking in the health care arena leads health professionals to view patients as consumers. Overtly, health professionals define consumers as people who are able to make their own decisions about the care they receive, express opinions about the care and evaluate the care, provided they are well enough to do so and wish to do so. This, it seems, is what health professionals aspire to, and it appears to be a simple enough task. However, literature within Australia and elsewhere shows that consumerism is very much a concept of tokenism or rhetoric with little action (Payle 1998). It is like saying: Is utopia attainable?

Parson's concept (Parsons 1957) of the sick role, espoused half a century ago, has long been dispensed with by health professionals and yet we are far from the ideal of patients as consumers (at least by those who wish to) in our hospitals. One feasible explanation is that the rhetoric of consumerism is clearly undercut by the realities of the practice setting. Further expansion on this is warranted here. The operational definition of consumer, as we know it, embraces the notion of empowerment for the user of a service or the purchaser of a product. In simple terms, if consumers do not like what they have bought, they are entitled to return the product and expect a refund, as per the Fair Trading policy. Similarly, if they are not satisfied with a service such as household goods repair, then they are within their right to withhold payment until the job is done to their satisfaction. However, health care as a product tends to fit outside the consumer model, because consumers of health care, especially in hospitals, do not have the same opportunity to demand a refund if their care is less than satisfactory or if they have not been consulted about their care. One cannot take poor or unsatisfactory health care back for a refund, and besides, patients as consumers are sometimes too sick to complain and often feel that they do not have any power to act.

Hospitals are complex bureaucratic organizations with ever-shrinking budgets. Is it enough rationalization to say that economic constraints with all its parameters is incongruent with the ideal of patient consumerism? Certainly not, and to think so will be naïve. The findings of a qualitative grounded theory study that I conducted will be used in this chapter in an attempt to throw some light on the impact of consumerism in hospitals. As I will show, the ideal of consumerism in health care, at least in the hospital context, is undermined by the reality of what actually happens in practice.

The study, undertaken in Perth, Western Australia, in 1998, was based on in-depth interviews with 33 nurses, 32 patients and 144 hours of observation in the hospitals. Four acute care hospitals, public and private, took part in the study. For a full account of the study's methodology, the reader is directed to Henderson (1998). With respect to consumerism within the hospital context, it is apparent that, at one end, there are hospital adminis-trators who, through no fault of their own, are forced to become 'bean counters'. Their role has become one of managing the shrinking health dollar and keeping the hospitals afloat. In the middle, are the majority of health professionals with their entrenched belief that they serve patients best by being the primary decision-makers in providing health care, leaving little room for consumer input. Lastly, we have the new breed of baby-boomer consumers (i.e. those born between 1945 and 1965) who are better informed about health issues and who are likely to expect interaction and indeed demand that their voices be heard. This is reflected in research conducted by Annandale (1996). In this UK study, nurses and midwives found consumers to be more aware of their rights and entitlement, to voice their expectations, and to seek information from them (1996: 422). The emphasis on the Patient's Charter (Walsh 1994), the media, and newspaper reports were perceived to contribute to this apparent increase in consumer demand. We can also add the Internet to this list. In Australia, the majority of homes have computers and more and more people are seeking information on the Net.

The findings of my study highlight that neo-liberal views on consumerism have come face to face with issues that constitute the backdrop to health care. These include economic constraints, the dominance of medical culture in hospitals and the presence of technology that is burgeoning at an alarming rate. To top this, the recently introduced Australian government's policy urging people to take out private health insurance has added to consumer expectations that 'if I am paying for it, I am going to get the care that I want'.

Australia, as a small multi-cultural society, has long been held as a testing ground for the marketing of techniques and products by companies world wide. Therefore, any information about consumer reactions (again from those who wish to take up the role of consumers) within the Australian health care arena presents a unique microcosm that is likely to parallel consumer status in other parts of the developed world. Thus, the reader is reminded that the findings presented here may have contextual relevance that may be applicable across hospital environments on a broader level. As well, patients' experiences of consumerism reported in this chapter are from the perspective of those patients who wished to have a say in what happens to them in hospital. It is important to bear in mind that not all patients wanted to take up the role of consumers, although these were in the minority in this study.

Consumerism and economic constraints

Both patients' and nurses' comments in my study demonstrate the contextual difficulties that patients may face in their enactment of consumerism in the hospital setting. It is apparent from the study that economic constraints may have contributed to this situation, as highlighted by these comments:

> They change shifts so often, you would be lucky to have the same nurses twice ... some [nurses] are nice and will ask for your opinion but others will come in and tell you what to do and cut out on you ... it can be frustrating.
>
> (Patient)

> With the government cutbacks on money and employment opportunity, I find that quite often our shift has been cut so you find yourself racing through, trying to get everything done before your shift is completed ... this leaves little time to do things like giving information to patients, which they need to become involved as consumers.
>
> (Nurse)

In Australia, the health care system has been subjected to several changes in recent times, especially in the area of funds allocation. The Commonwealth Government distributes substantial funds to the States for health care. However, according to Burns (1998) and Witham (1996), the States have withdrawn, for other use, large amounts of funds allocated for hospitals, leaving them short of funds. Witham (1996) further claims that this clawback by the States has put hospitals under enormous pressure to cut costs to enable them to manage their reduced budgets. Cuthbert et al. (1992) concur with the above authors, claiming that once the States have been allocated their funds by the Commonwealth Government, they are free to use the funds as they deem necessary. For example, Witham (1996) reports that, since 1988, the States have withdrawn about $700 million from their hospital budgets, forcing hospitals to cut costs. These cutbacks have resulted in hospitals having to undergo vast restructuring (O'Connell 1997; Henderson 1998; Paradies 1996). To cope with the limited funds available, hospital administrators possibly have no choice but to become 'bean counters', thus embracing the bureaucratic view of consumerism based on controlling costs, patient outcomes and staff efficiency.

A major consequence of restructuring is the reduction in permanent nursing staff being employed by hospitals, frequently leaving wards short-staffed. As a result of these staff shortages, there has been an increase in the number of private agency nurses being employed by hospitals (O'Connell 1997). So how has this affected patient consumerism? Nurses and patients in the study reported that there was lack of continuity of care. In other words, care has become fragmented. The fragmentation in care effectively prevented the development of mutual respect and interaction between nurses and patients. Both patients and nurses believed that the fulfilment of the consumerist ideal is facilitated by positive nurse–patient relationships. Additionally, nurses and patients perceive that there are not enough nurses to cope with the demands of the wards and to meet all patients' needs, including giving them choice. This concurs with the findings of other Australian studies (Irurita 1993; O'Connell 1997; Williams 1996). The nurses in Williams' (1996) study in particular, claim that they are not always able to engage in positive nurse–patient interactions because they are short staffed.

Some nurses and patients in my study claimed that staff shortages inhib-ited or modified the fulfilment of the role of consumers by patients. The nurses stated that they had insufficient time to provide patients with infor-mation and to sit and talk with them, in order to get to know them beyond their medical diagnosis. The nurses perceived that patients needed to be fully informed if they are to make their own decision about their care, in order to behave as expected of consumers. Some nurses agreed that at times they did have the time to provide information and to educate patients. However, they voiced concern that, due to the staff shortages, they were unable 'consis-tently' to provide patients with needed information and to invite them to have choice. This situation contradicts the essence of consumerism because unless patients are given information and choice, they cannot be empowered to act as consumers. The nurses claimed that they were sometimes called away to work in another ward in the middle of their shift if their ward was not busy. This effectively prevented information sharing and patient teaching, which according to these nurses is usually only possible when the wards are quiet. For example:

> We are short staffed and we don't have the time to do a lot of things like patient teaching or sit and give them [patients] information ... maybe it is less people power around the place ... bells and phones ringing!
>
> (Nurse)

> ... only through trust and knowing you that patients will feel comfort-able about telling you what they are able to do, what they can't do and feel free to make their own decisions about their care ... but when your back is to the wall and you are under so much pressure, I mean it is easier if you don't ask for their opinion.
>
> (Nurse)

It is evident from the study that some nurses believe that patients should be consumers, through working with them as partners, but feel that this is incompatible with the overall goals of the hospital management structure. The introduction of Diagnosis Related Group (a system in which acute care patients are classified into medical diagnosis) and Casemix funding (a costing formula that pertains to the mix of patients treated in specific wards) where hospitals are paid prospectively for services rendered, mean that hospitals are eager to discharge patients early in order to process as many patients as possible within a given period of time. One can almost liken a hospital to a 'body-processing plant' where the greater the turnover of patients, the greater the financial remuneration for the hospital. It is no surprise therefore, that several Australian hospitals have opted for the early discharge programme. This leaves little time for patients and nurses to interact and work as partners:

> Patients are short-term stays as they are only in for 3 or 4 days ... um, you know them more in what they are in for than who they are in terms of a person, what their wants and needs are ... I think the nursing care is congested with Casemix for example, on day 1, patients should be doing this, this and this; day 2, this and this; day 3 they are going home ... it is all predetermined with clinical pathways ... with early discharge, we don't have much contact with patients to work with them.
>
> (Nurse)

Nursing care being congested means that all care has to be rushed through within a time frame, in keeping with the use of clinical pathways which are part of the DRG classification system. Clinical pathways are interdisciplinary plans of care that outline the optimal sequencing and timing of interventions for patients with a specific diagnosis, procedure or symptom (Ignatavicius and Hausman 1995). Moreover, non-medical aspects of care, such as sharing information with patients and talking with patients to get to know them as people and their capabilities, are difficult to achieve. Greenwood and King (1995) state that an Australian study into nurses' clinical judgement when clinical pathways are used, show that its use hinders nurses from providing care that involves patient input. They add that clinical pathways emphasize physical care with little regard for care that is patient focused. Categorically, the authors suggest that clinical pathways have arisen as a consequence of economic rationalism. Overall, the management of the hospital is said to be only interested in cost cutting and at times is prepared to sacrifice quality patient care in the name of economic rationalism. This concurs with George and Davis (2000) who state that the need to cut costs in Australian hospitals has resulted in administrators being more interested in input costs than in patient outcomes. Hence, the public's perception of administrators as 'bean counters'.

It may be said with some confidence, therefore, that the early discharge programme adopted by Australian hospitals is an integral part of hospital administrators stretching the health dollar. As noted in an Australian Institute of Health and Welfare report, the average length of stay for acute care hospital patients, both public and private, is steadily decreasing (Nursing Review 1997: 4). As patients' length of stay decreases, the amount of contact that nurses have with patients also decreases. This means that nurses have less time to get to know patients' capabilities and opinions about their care so that they can invite appropriate input (Henderson 1997).

So what is the impact of early discharge on patients as consumers? In my study, for patients, early discharge meant that they were initially too sick to make decisions about their care. By the time they were well enough to do so they were already discharged. To put it in another way, for some patients, there were no opportunities for the fulfilment of the ideal role of the consumer. For example:

> The patient turnover is high on this ward, they [patients] are coming and going all the time ... they are quite sick immediately post-op and you are kept busy doing physical care ... by the time they are ready to be involved, they are discharged but first you need to find out where patients are coming from and you can't do this always because they are too sick, so you tend to direct them which may not suit the patient.
>
> (Nurse)

The above nurse's comment was validated by field observations. Due to the early discharge programme and subsequent high patient turnover, permanent nurses on the wards were constantly faced with caring for newly admitted patients. These patients were observed to be sicker and required more physical care. In other words, the nurses' time was taken up in ensuring the stability of patients' vital signs and physical well-being, leaving them little time to offer choices to patients. It was not uncommon for patients to be cared for by as many as ten nurses within a four-day hospital stay, for instance:

> I think one thing in Australia I've noticed about is that because we don't have primary nursing and we are short staffed, it is difficult for patients to have any worthwhile input ... you see, one nurse may be admitting them and the next day somebody else is looking after them and the next day there might be somebody else again; it lacks continuity ... patients cannot identify with the same nurse, it is quite fragmented really.
>
> (Nurse)

The lack of continuity had also prevented patients from having input into their care as patients did not have the same nurses to initiate any negotiation with them about their care. Some nurses also gave them conflicting instructions, as indicated below:

> I am not the sort of person who picks, picks, and picks but it has been a bit frustrating with different nurses telling you different things ... you sort of think, what am I supposed to do? ... like I have been told to keep my leg up on a pillow by one nurse and to keep it level by another nurse ... also you can't tell them [nurses] anything because you don't see the same nurse twice.
>
> (Patient)

Patients commented that the early discharge programme took their choice away:

> The nurses seem to put everything into a little slot to get through their work ... they have their set duties ... it is beneficial for them but not for patients ... they take away your choice like after my haemorrhoid operation, I wanted to stay in hospital until I had my bowels working again but the nurse said I had to go home.
>
> (Patient)

Concern was expressed by some nurses that they would have involved patients in their own care more if they had continuity of care and patients were in hospital for a longer period of time. The nurses explained that they need time and patients need to be well enough before they can become aware of where the other was 'coming from'. This was considered to be important for negotiations to occur between the dyad. Given these circumstances, can it be argued that consumerism beyond a rhetoric is not achievable in acute care hospitals? To go one step further, can we settle for consumerism being better placed in an extended care type of health care setting where patients are not acutely ill and the stay is longer?

Culture of medical dominance

Cahill (1998) reports on doctors' and nurses' attitudes to consumer involvement in care. In reviewing the relevant literature on patient participation, Cahill writes that doctors' and nurses' views on the value of patient involvement in care are varied and that consumerism as an approach to care has neither been rejected nor embraced as a panacea by health professionals (1998: 10). There is literature and research from medical sociology that demonstrate that some patients still prefer to enact the traditional passive role (Biley 1992), despite them being well enough to adopt a consumerist stance. The predominant reason indicated in the literature is one of lack of medical knowledge and information on the part of the patient. This begs the question of why health professionals are far from strident in coming forward and giving information to patients.

In my study, nurses claimed that they lacked time in their busy schedule to give patients adequate information. However, at a deeper level, it was revealed that nurses were reluctant to relinquish their power to patients. It was evident that nurses worked in an environment that supported the culture of medical dominance. Even though this dominance was not obviously noticeable, it nevertheless was perceived to be present by some nurses and patients. Very few nurses were observed to share their power and knowledge with patients. The majority tended to hold on to their power by giving only minimal information to patients. The information that was given also tended to be procedural in nature with nurses using medical jargon. The following comment shows that nurses have power and knowledge:

> The patient relinquishes power ... the nurse assumes power – not power ... power is a silly word, I don't know if I like 'power' ... I suppose on the whole a lot of nurses are almost a bossy breed ... we have quite a few of the staff with that attitude. I suppose we want them [patients] to succumb to whatever we want them to do and we use terminology that they don't understand, that is alien to them.
>
> (Nurse)

A few patients expressed concern that they did not have the power to voice their opinions in hospital. This was perceived to be due to lack of medical knowledge as shown below:

> You have to do as they [nurses] tell you, otherwise they could give you the wrong medicine or something and then what could you do, you are really in their hands! ... you are not told anything!
>
> (Patient)

> I didn't want to say anything or do anything without their permission [nurses] ... I felt that I have to do as they told me to because I am a patient and they know what is best for me ... I couldn't voice my opinion because I didn't know much about my surgery and they didn't tell me.
>
> (Patient)

Beck (1997) explains that there are implicit power differentials between patients and health professionals as indicated by certain perpetuated behaviours between the two groups. This is despite society's trend to push for a consumerist approach to health care (Beck and Regan 1995; Smith-Dupre and Beck 1996). Beck is supported by May (1992) who says that despite nurses placing emphasis on a participatory approach to care, nurses make no attempt to democratize the unequal power relationship that exists between them and patients. According to May, nurses retain their power by controlling the nature of interactions between them and patients and by avoiding making reciprocal disclosures to patients. Lawler (1991) adds that nurses continue to exercise power similar to that of doctors over patients by withholding information from them. The above views are also reflected in my own study, as shown below:

> I don't volunteer medical or treatment information to patients unless they ask and some do ... I don't care what anybody says ... patients cooperate in hospital, we give them the information so they can decide about basic things like their shower ... why bother coming into hospital if they [patients] want to make treatment and medical decisions ... I always explain what I am doing to them and that should be enough ... we know best anyway for their recovery.
>
> (Nurse)

The lack of knowledge and information places patients in a disadvantaged position in that they are not able to make informed decisions about their care (Avis 1994; Irvine 1996). As a result, patients have a tendency to defer to professional opinion. Nurses' perception that they know best is confirmed by McCormack (1993) who states that nurses often fall into the rhetoric of thinking and believing that they are doing the right thing for patients which can affect patient input. Some nurses, and indeed some patients in this study, really believed that patients do not have expert medical knowledge to contribute in a partnership model of care.

> They [doctors and nurses] are trained, and in my opinion should have an overriding say ... they should decide about my treatments as I know absolutely nothing about my medical situation unless they explain everything in lay terms.
>
> (Patient)

Several nurses commented that they needed to act as advocates for patients if they are to be consumers. However, they expressed concern that this was not always possible due to ramifications from medical staff. The nurses claimed that they did not feel comfortable in encouraging patients to seek, or ask about, alternative modes of treatment because it meant that they were going against the doctor's planned treatment for the patient. The nurses felt powerless with regard to going against the doctor's decision:

> It is hard when the doctor wants to send the patient for a procedure but the patient does not want to have it done, for example, chemotherapy ... they'd rather have palliative care and die with dignity ... you can't interfere

because you feel you are overstepping the line and you could be hauled over the coals by administration ... sometimes I think we are only able to give lip service to our role as patient advocates.

(Informal nurse interview)

The nurses had no difficulty in stating that it was the doctors' responsibility to give patients information about their medical condition. They felt strongly, however, that doctors needed to provide comprehensive information to patients and not just inform them about the procedures that they had scheduled for them. Furthermore, the nurses expressed concern that some doctors were not providing patients with all the information to enable them to make their own decisions. The nurses claimed that they were unable to speak to some doctors about not giving adequate information to patients because they felt that doctors do not always listen.

We are supposed to be patient advocates and you know, we have the right to say to the doctor, 'You have just walked in here and you have said this and this and the patient is very anxious and upset, I would like you to sit down and discuss what exactly you are going to do to him [patient] ... he is absolutely terrified and you haven't helped matters by going in there and walking out as if he is just a piece of meat that you are going to cut open and go home', but nurses don't have the power ... not all doctors will listen and some have an attitude towards nurses ...

(Nurse)

The nurses also perceived that they should be more proactive in fulfilling their advocacy role if they are to promote consumerism. They explained that sometimes it is much easier for some nurses to blame the doctors than to advocate for patients. Advocating for patients means taking on more responsibility. The above nurse claimed that some nurses were of the view that they should follow doctors' orders, and provide the treatment that was ordered for them, without allowing patients any say in that ordered treatment. These nurses were not perceived by other nurses to be concerned about empowering patients. Instead they were concerned about pleasing the doctors and encouraged patients to follow the doctors' orders:

I think a lot of nurses don't even think about the empowering aspect of care ... it's a term that they never ever have learned or it has never been in their minds ... like I said earlier, some people should never have become nurses ... I think they come into nursing to meet nice young doctors ... you can tell the way these young girls [nurses] flutter their eyelashes at the doctor and hang on every word he says without thinking about the patient's needs.

(Informal nurse interview)

The nurses explained that being an advocate involved taking risks like going against the medical profession which could have detrimental effects on them. This opinion was prevalent in ward areas where the nurses perceived that they would not receive adequate support from nursing administration should they be challenged by doctors while advocating for patients.

> Sometimes you see things happen to patients that you feel you should say something to the doctor about but that will be putting your neck in a noose ... undermine a doctor?, no way, especially one who makes money for the hospital ... I realize of course that I should have the right to say it but I might as well not ... to be a realist, I realize that if I did say anything my arse will be grass and I will be out the door that fast.
>
> (Nurse)

In support of this, Becker (1986) states that being an advocate is sometimes risky for nurses. The author claims that nurses may lose their jobs if they are perceived to be trouble-makers by the nursing hierarchy because they went against the doctor's decision and advocated for the patient. This, according to the author, is especially true for situations where nurses have supported patients to seek alternative modes of treatment in their zest to promote self-determination in them. Furthermore, Becker reports that the fear of losing their positions has sometimes rendered nurses to be passive advocates, which involves supporting patients only within the boundaries of the norms and rules as set out by those in authority, namely the medical staff. Kubsch (1996) concurs with Becker, stating that in reality the hospital culture is very much dominated by the medical staff and that nurses' responsibilities inherently involve following medical orders.

In relation to power and knowledge in the context of health and illness, much of Foucault's work (1975; 1980; 1991) has been quoted. Foucault challenges the objectifying of the patient as a body that needs surveillance and monitoring by medical personnel. The term 'clinical gaze' designates the situation whereby health professionals continue to treat patients as bodies with little concern for their rights as individuals. According to May (1992) the subjectification of patients by nurses can increase patients' control and empower them. However, nurses must first realize that health care in Australia, as in other countries, is inextricably connected with power and politics. Nurses must be empowered themselves to overcome the restraints of their own environment before they can empower patients. Watts (1990: 41) states that it is timely that nurses, through political involvement and confrontation with power holders, reclaim their right and worth in the health care arena in Australia and elsewhere. Only then can nurses feel empowered to be able to empower patients.

Presence of technology

The study revealed that the presence of technology sometimes inhibited patients from being consumers in hospital. McKinlay's (1979) argument that technology takes centre stage in health care over two decades ago, is still valid today. Field observations showed that complex equipment is widely used in hospitals, and nurses have to work frequently with technology and be capable of handling machinery in order to provide direct patient care. While nurses acknowledge the benefits of using medical equipment, they point out that learning how to use the machines is time consuming and stressful. This further reduces nurses' time for interaction with patients and promoting their input:

> It is the hospital environment, there are so many gadgets that you have to be familiar with like special pumps and monitors which take up the time ... they are things that require a lot of time to make sure they [pumps, machinery, monitors] are running properly ... doesn't leave much time to be with patients and involve them in care ... pretty stressful too.
>
> (Nurse)

The concern about being stressed when working with unfamiliar equipment is supported by McConnell and Fletcher's (1995) study. Their findings show that the majority of the 142 nurses studied had to learn the equipment using the manual or through other nurses. A third of these nurses also suffered stress. Together with other writers (McConnell, Fletcher and Nissan 1993; McConnell and Nissan 1993), McConnell reports that the use of medical equipment is a double-edged sword which can either enhance or inhibit care that is patient focused. Factors, such as nurses' level of proficiency, knowledge and understanding, warrant consideration when it comes to the use of medical equipment.

Some nurses in my study explained that looking after machines sometimes took precedence over caring for patients in a manner that promoted patient involvement. The nurses claimed that the operation of machines took up so much of their time during the shift that they had no time left to work with patients. They added that, because they had insufficient time with patients, they had no option but to revert to task-oriented care. This was in direct conflict with their beliefs that patients should be consumers:

> Really, I would like to get patients involved in their care but I find I don't have the time ... getting patients to participate takes time ... patients can be quite slow ... I know I have a responsibility to make sure the machine is working correctly so I find myself working with the machine more, instead of the patient.
>
> (Informal nurse interview)

While some nurses expressed concern about not having the time to work with patients because of machinery, other nurses were observed to only have regular contact with patients who had machinery attached to them. It was interesting to observe these nurses going immediately to the patient's bedside whenever the machine's alarm sounded. However, when patients with machines rang the call bell, these nurses did not respond as quickly, as demonstrated by these field notes:

> The patient had a PCA [patient controlled analgesia] machine attached. The patient had two drains and an ordinary intravenous line. He had an oxygen mask on. Suddenly, the alarm on the PCA machine went and within minutes the nurse was in. She fiddled with the machine without looking at the patient or saying anything to him. When the alarm stopped, the nurse left the room. A few minutes later, the patient rang the bell and waited. Ten minutes passed before the patient rang again. Five minutes later, the nurse came into the room, 'What do you want Mr X?' asked the nurse. 'I want the bowl, I feel sick' to which the nurse said, 'Hang on, I will go and get you one' and left the room. A few minutes later, she came back with the bowl but the patient had already started to vomit.
>
> (Field notes)

A few patients said that machines had become the interface between patients and nurses instead of the nurse being the interface between machines and patients. They expressed concern that some nurses had become over-reliant on machines to the detriment of maintaining patient contact and finding out what patients can and cannot do in terms of having a say in their care. Moreover, the patients claimed that some nurses depended on the machines to assess their progress rather than to assess them physically or take note of what patients said about their well-being:

> The patient turned to the nurse while she was sorting out the machine's alarm and said, 'I don't feel so good' to which the nurse replied, 'After I have fixed the knob, you will be ok' and continued to fiddle with the machine instead of listening to the patient. The patient collapsed and needed emergency fluid replacement.
>
> (Field notes)

> Sometimes, I am sure nurses must think machines keep patients alive ... there is this attitude that if the machine is working then the patient is cared for.
>
> (Informal patient interview)

Other patients claimed that they were hindered from taking a proactive role in their care because they were concerned about doing harm to the equipment. The patients said that they lacked sufficient information because no one had explained about the equipment to them. Hence, they were frightened to do anything, in case they caused problems for themselves through mishandling the equipment:

> You have all these tubes and things and you are scared to move or do anything in case you do yourself an injury ... might pull something out and end up in hospital longer ... so it is best to wait for the nurse to come and take you to the shower ... she [nurse] will know what to do.
>
> (Patient)

Conclusion

In conclusion, I would like to remind the reader that the intention of this chapter has not been to advocate for or against consumerism, but rather to examine the factors limiting the operation of consumerism in the hospital context. As I have shown, the major factors that inhibited consumerism in the hospital context have been economic constraints, medical dominance and the presence of technology. While the findings of my study can only be applied to the specific context in which it was conducted, they nevertheless demonstrate that consumerism remains at only the conceptual level, with a long way to go before becoming operational in the practice setting. At this point, I wonder whether consumerism can ever be more than rhetoric, given the present hospital environment that I have described. I say this for the following reasons. As I see it, economic constraints are largely outside the scope of health professionals to change, as they are influenced and controlled by world economic pressures, the national economic strength, and the social and political policies of the government of the day. With regards to the culture of medical dominance, unless doctors and nurses are willing to relinquish some of their assumed powers to patients, the ideals underlying consumerism are unlikely to be realized. As demonstrated in my study, by depriving the patient of vital information including treatment options, doctors and nurses can only bring about the fruition of the self-fulfilling prophesy of health professionals, that is, patients prefer not to get involved. This chapter has shown that the greatest problem facing nurses is the lack of time available to invite patient involvement. This has been brought about by staff shortages and nurses having to learn how to use technology and machines. As indicated in the chapter, hospitals are increasingly using technology. Can one, therefore, be so bold as to argue that machines are being used more and more as robot nurses, that is, as simply a replacement for human labour? More specifically, have nurses come to rely on machines as an inter-phase between themselves and the patient rather than regarding the machines as an extension of themselves? These are some of the questions that need addressing by the nursing profession. Finally, the question about consumerism in hospital needs to be debated in the context of its limitations. The chapter has shown that patients cannot be true consumers in hospital because of various constraints, and health professionals have a long way to go before they can claim that patients are able to participate in the ways implied by the rhetoric of consumerism.

References

Annandale, E. (1996) 'Working on the front line: risk culture and nursing in the new NHS', *The Sociological Review*, 44, 3: 416–51.

Avis, M. (1994) 'Choice cuts: an exploratory study of patients' views about participation in decision-making in a day surgery unit', *International Journal of Nursing Studies*, 31, 3: 289–98.

Beck, C.S. (1997) 'How can I put this? Exaggerated self-disparagement as alignment strategy during problematic disclosures by patients to doctors', *Qualitative Health Research*, 7, 4: 487–503.

Beck, C. and Regan, S.L. (1995) 'The impact of relational activities on the accomplishment of practitioner and patient goals in the gynaecologic examination', in G. Kreps and D. O'Hair (eds) *Communication and Health Outcomes*, Cresskill, NJ: Hampton, pp. 73–86.

Becker, P.H. (1986) 'Advocacy in nursing: perils and possibilities', *Holistic Nursing Practice*, 11, 1: 54–63.

Biley, F.C. (1992) 'Some determinants that affect patient participation in decision making about nursing care', *Journal of Advanced Nursing*, 17, 41: 4–421.

Burns, A. (1998) 'States spend $27 per head less on hospitals', *The West Australian*, 7 April: 10.

Cahill, J. (1998) 'Patient participation: a review of the literature', *Journal of Clinical Nursing*, 7, 2: 119–28.

Cuthbert, M., Duffield, C. and Hope, J. (1992) *Management in Nursing*, Sydney: Harcourt Brace Jovanovich.

Foucault, M. (1975) *The Birth of the Clinic: An Archaeology of Medical Perception*, New York: Vintage Books.

—— (1980) 'Body/power', in C. Gordon (ed.) *Power/Knowledge: Selected Interviews and Other Writings by Michel Foucault, 1972–1977*, New York: Pantheon.

—— (1991) 'The politics of health in the eighteenth century', in P. Rainbow (ed.) *The Foucault Reader*, London: Penguin.

George, J. and Davis, A. (2000) *States of Health: Health and Illness in Australia* (3rd edn), Sydney: Longman.

Greenwood, J. and King, M. (1995) 'Nursing orthopaedic patients: profoundly absorbing work', in G. Gray and R. Pratt (eds) *Issues in Nursing 5*, Melbourne: Churchill Livingstone.

Henderson, S. (1997) 'Knowing the patient and the impact on patient participation: a grounded theory study', *International Journal of Nursing Practice*, 3, 2: 111–18.

—— (1998) *The phenomenon of patient participation in their nursing care: a grounded theory study*, unpublished PhD thesis, Curtin University of Technology.

Ignatavicius, D.D. and Hausman, K.A. (1995) *Clinical Pathways for Collaborative Practice*, Sydney: W.B. Saunders Company.

Irurita, V. (1993) *From Person to Patient: Nursing Care from the Patient's Perspective*, Western Australia: Curtin University of Technology.

Irvine, R. (1996) 'Losing patients: health care consumers, power and sociological change', in C. Grbich (ed.) *Health in Australia: Sociological Concepts and Issues*, Sydney: Prentice Hall, pp. 191–214.

Kubsch, S.M. (1996) 'Conflict, enactment, empowerment: conditions of independent therapeutic nursing intervention', *Journal of Advanced Nursing*, 23: 192–200.

Lawler, J. (1991) *Behind the Scenes: Nursing, Somology and the Problem of the Body*, Melbourne: Churchill Livingstone.

May, C. (1992) 'Nursing work, nurses' knowledge, and the subjectification of the patient', *Sociology of Health and Illness*, 14, 4: 473–87.

McConnell, E.A. and Fletcher, J. (1995) 'Agency registered nurse use of medical equipment: an Australian perspective', *International Journal of Nursing Studies*, 32, 2: 149–61.

McConnell, E.A., Fletcher, J. and Nissan, J.H. (1993) 'A comparison of Australian and American registered nurses' use of life-sustaining medical devices in critical care and high-dependency units', *Heart and Lung*, 22: 421–7.

McConnell, E.A. and Nissan, J.H. (1993) 'The use of medical equipment by Australian registered nurses', *Journal of Clinical Nursing*, 2: 341–8.

McCormack, B. (1993) 'How to promote quality of care and preserve patient autonomy', *British Journal of Nursing*, 2, 6: 338–40.

McKinlay, J.B. (1979) 'Epidemiological and political determinants of social policies regarding the public health', *Social Science and Medicine*, 13A: 541–8.

Nursing Review (1997) *More Admissions, Shorter Stays*, College of Nursing, Australia, September, p. 4.

O'Connell, B. (1997) *A grounded theory study of the clinical use of the nursing process within selected hospital settings*, unpublished PhD thesis, Curtin University of Technology.

Paradies, P. (1996) 'Brisbane faces acute shortages', *Nursing Review*, College of Nursing, Australia, October, p. 19.

Parsons, T. (1957) *The Social System*, Glencoe, IL: Free Press.

Payle, J.F. (1998) 'Health professionals' views on patient participation: treading a fine line', Paper presented at the 4th Qualitative Research Conference, Vancouver, Canada.

Smith-Dupre, A. and Beck, C. (1996) 'Enabling patients and physicians to pursue multiple goals in health care encounters: a case study', *Health Communication*, 8: 73–90.

Walsh, K. (1994) 'Citizens, charters and contracts', in R. Keat, N. Whitely and N. Abercrombie (eds) *The Authority of the Consumer*, London: Routledge.

Watts, R.J. (1990) 'Democratization of health care: challenge for nursing', *Advances in Nursing Science*, 12, 2: 37–46.

Williams, A.M. (1996) *The delivery of quality nursing care: a grounded theory study of the nurse's perspective*, unpublished Masters thesis, Curtin University of Technology.

Witham, H. (1996) 'Australian health care faces crisis as nurses bail out', *Nursing Review*, Royal Nursing College, Australia, January, p. 3.

Chapter 7

Consumerism and mental health care in a culturally diverse society

Alan Petersen, Renata Kokanovic and Susan Hansen

This chapter[1] examines the extent to which consumerism has come to inform mental health care policy, and the limitations and implications of the consumerism model a culturally diverse society. Mental illness and mental health care are issues that directly or indirectly affect all of us. At some point in our lives, we are likely to feel depressed or be described as 'mentally disordered'. At the very least, we will know someone who has come into direct contact with the mental health care system. During such times, discussions about care and the adequacy of therapeutic options are likely to come to the fore. Such discussions are often framed in both the policy- and the personal-realm by the language of consumerism, by which the 'costs' associated with mental illness and its care are considered substantial, for affected individuals and for the community as a whole. These 'costs' include both economic expenses (e.g. medical treatment and lost income through time off work by those diagnosed as 'ill' and those who offer their unpaid assistance), social costs (disruption to relationships) and emotional costs (the resulting distress for all concerned). It is for these reasons that mental health problems have increasingly been the focus of public policy. However, although an ethos of consumerism is increasingly evident in mental health care – in the conduct and evaluation of mental health services – few policy-makers question the applicability, or acknowledge the limits of, the consumerism model.

Furthermore, despite the development of diverse critical perspectives on 'mental illness' – to which sociology, social anthropology and critical psychology have contributed significantly – in the 'practical' realm of mental health services, alternatives to the disease or deficit model are seldom evident in practice (Mechanic 1999). The high value accorded to psychiatry – which operates according to the disease model, and which promotes pharmaceutical treatment – and the growing influence of 'evidence-based practice' (EBP), has meant that the less quantifiable or 'messy' dimensions of 'mental health care' have been largely neglected. The EBP model has proved attractive to health policy-makers as it appeals to the imperative to regulate the cost of services. However, critics note that evidence-based approaches are often restricted by their emphasis on a professional definition of 'treatment effectiveness', and seldom take account of the experiences and views of service-users – or 'consumers' – and their families in formulating such 'evidence' (Pilgrim and Rogers 1999).

The neglect of the unpaid carer perspective in the study of 'mental illness' and mental health seems odd given the growing emphasis on consumerism in health and welfare, and the devolution of responsibility for caring work, i.e. 'care in the community' (see, e.g., Hugman 1994). In the mental health field, the focus on 'care in the community' has gone hand in hand with de-institutionalization – or the practice of 'emptying' residential psychiatric institutions. De-institutionalization appears to be a universal feature of contemporary mental health care systems, although it is proceeding at an uneven pace throughout the world (Lefley 1999: 580). Commentators argue that governments have initiated policies of de-institutionalization in their efforts to reduce the costs associated with maintaining psychiatric institutions (e.g. Mulvaney 1994). In Australia, the number of psychiatric hospital beds declined from 281 beds per 100,000 people in the early 1960s to 40 beds per 100,000 people in the 1990s (National Health Strategy 1993). Over this period there was a corresponding shift in the terminology used to describe the identities of affected persons: those who left psychiatric hospitals (the 'mental patients') were increasingly addressed as 'clients' in the community mental health system. This implied a degree of freedom not available to hospitalized patients (Kaufmann 1999: 495). However, despite the widely held assumption that 'care in the community' is 'empowering' for 'consumers'/'clients', what evidence exists suggests major inadequacies with de-institutionalization. For de-institutionalized 'clients', these may include social isolation and discrimination, lack of social and economic support and opportunities, and the lack of availability and/or fragmentation and poor coordination of mental health and social services (Mulvaney 1998: 262–3). Access to appropriate accommodation is fundamental for health and well-being (Marmot 1999). Yet research in the UK, the US and Australia has identified a range of housing problems that tend to be faced by de-institutionalized mental health service 'consumers'.

The problems experienced by people diagnosed with mental illness stem from a combination of financial constraints, and inappropriate and poor-quality housing stock (Mulvaney 1998: 263–8). In some jurisdictions, the 'community treatment order' – under which patients live in the community and are supervised by medical practitioners – has been used by policy-makers as a means to justify the 'right' to control people who are described as 'potentially dangerous and criminal' (Mulvaney 1994). In such cases, it is evident that some party other than the 'consumer' is being served under those sections of mental health legislation that accord professionals the right to dictate treatment interventions against a 'consumer's' wishes. Certainly, if a person is confined in the absence of a trial, and they are 'treated' in the absence of consent, it is difficult to describe them as informed 'customers' or 'clients' (Pilgrim and Rogers 1999). In such circumstances, the logic of the alternative nomenclature favoured by the psychiatric service users' movement – of 'recipients' or 'survivors' – becomes more readily apparent. As neo-liberal policies increasingly de-emphasize government responsibility for the provision of services in favour of a regulatory role, health care systems have assumed a corresponding 'consumer' or 'client' orientation. With this shift in focus, it is imperative to explore the impact of the philosophy of consumerism, and its related practices, on the lives and relationships of the 'consumers'/'clients' – or 'recipients'/'survivors' – of mental health care services.

The applicability and value of the consumerism model to mental health care, and to health care more generally, is highly questionable. First, it needs to be asked under what conditions are people able to behave as 'good' consumers of mental health services – that is, according to the principle of consumer sovereignty in which the consumers are seen as the best judge of their own welfare (Shackley and Ryan 1994: 522). Who are the assumed 'consumers' anyway, and what exactly are they 'consuming'? Further, and in relation to issues of access, equity and appropriateness, what efforts are made to involve 'consumers' in the decisions that affect them? Are the needs of all 'consumers' being adequately met in a culturally appropriate manner? Do people have access to the information and services that will best assist them in their caring role? What do people say will assist them in this regard? The investigation of such questions is crucial to the evaluation of the impact of recent changes in policy direction.

Although the manifestation of consumerism would seem to vary considerably between countries – with perhaps the US presenting the more extreme example of consumerism in practice – commentators have noted for diverse health care systems that the relationship between professionals and 'patients'/'clients' has shifted. Increasingly, health policy endorses the values of autonomous decision-making, self-reliance and the need for people to 'participate' actively in discussions and decisions about options and priorities – evident from, for example, the UK Government's document *The Health of the Nation* (Secretary of State for Health 1991). People are expected to exercise 'informed choice', to use information technology, to access information, to control their own health, and to consult professionals less than before (Smith 1997: 1496).

Despite similarities in the rhetoric of participation that now characterize health care policy in general and mental health care policy in particular, there are some crucial differences in the ways that these services tend to operate *in practice*. Consumers of mental health services are very differently positioned from consumers of other health services. However, these differences are often concealed by the similarities in the clinical classification systems, and in the language used to describe the 'needs' of consumers. Indeed, there are a number of problems that are particular to the appropriation of the consumer model by the mental health 'industry'. Firstly, the services actually 'provided' by this 'industry' vary enormously, and range from forced detention, and (in)voluntary electro-convulsive shock therapy, to voluntary attendance at 'talking therapy' sessions (Pilgrim and Rogers 1999). A variety of services are available between these extremes, and involve a blend of coercive and voluntary therapies. Notably, the element that separates these extremes is that of 'free choice' – generally seen as being a prerequisite for an 'informed consumer'.

The market model of health care, which assumes conditions of 'perfect' competition, where 'consumers' have 'perfect' knowledge and act free of the self-interested advice of suppliers, has been shown to be severely wanting. In the health care market-place, in which there is an asymmetry of information between 'buyers' and 'sellers', consumer sovereignty is likely to be very limited (Shackley and Ryan 1994: 524). Indeed, the knowledge of 'consumers' and that of (mental) health professionals is differently valued. 'Consumers' are vulnerable to exploitation by 'better-informed' providers who may recommend ineffective or inappropriate 'treatments'. Further, the informational asymmetry is likely to take a special form in health care in that it extends beyond the characteristics of the 'product' to the effect of the product on the user. Paradoxically, the rhetoric of consumerism is structured to enable providers to make decisions that override the expressed 'needs' of consumers. Commonsensical examples of the conditions under which such decisions are regarded as necessary tend to be drawn from the more 'serious' end of the health care scale. Here, 'consumers' with a life-threatening illness may be deemed not to be the best judge of their own interests, due to the gravity of the situation (Shackley and Ryan 1994: 525). Such decisions are justified along similar lines in the realm of mental health care, where the clinician's assessment of 'lack of insight' on the part of the consumer can effectively remove the capacity of the latter to make decisions about their own treatment.

Providers of mental health services, then, do not always act in a manner expected of 'good' 'producers' and 'sellers'. That is, they are likely either to not provide the services wanted by 'buyers', or to offer services that are far from 'user-friendly' in practice. Services are frequently insensitive to cultural and linguistic differences, and often fail to recognize cross-cultural differences in definitions of emotional well-being and in preferred approaches to treatment (Kokanovic et al. 2001). Service providers seem also not to appreciate the stigma that may follow the diagnosis of a mental illness – both for those so described and for their families (Pilgrim and Rogers 1999). The consumer model is then especially problematic for users of mental health services, at least in part because the stigma attached to 'mental illness' in many communities provides a powerful disincentive for people to actively seek information or help outside of their immediate family or community. Diagnostic labels such as 'schizophrenia' and 'depression' are likely to have negative consequences in people's daily lives – at the very least, persons so described may be treated differently across a wide range of situations, and excluded altogether from others.

Finally, the little empirical evidence that exists indicates that, in any case, people often do not act in accordance with the consumerism model. In other words, they do not behave as would be expected of 'good' consumers of health care. For example, people frequently do not exhibit information-seeking behaviour and may not want to exercise choice and be responsible for health care decisions, but instead prefer to place faith and trust in professionals to make the right decisions. That is, they would prefer to adhere to the traditional model of medicine, where the doctor is in charge and the patient is dependent. Although trust in medicine has waned somewhat, and is tempered by a measure of mistrust that limits its authority to its clinical domain, medical dominance remains a general feature of many health care systems (Daniel 1998). The extent to which people either defer to medical or psychological authority, or adhere to consumerist behaviour varies considerably. There is some evidence to suggest that elderly people, at least in some groups, may be less inclined and less 'able' than younger people to act in an 'ideal' consumer-oriented manner (Shackley and Ryan 1994: 532–6). Such behaviour is also, of course, culturally variable.

The issue of 'cultural competence'

Despite the increasing calls for policy-makers to become 'culturally competent' in health care – that is, to become culturally credible 'problem-solvers' (see Chin 2000) – 'consumers' from diverse cultures are seldom consulted in the development and evaluation of mental health services. Recent immigrants, whose first language is not that of the host country and who tend to be unfamiliar with local social structures, values and mores, may have their own equally valid understandings of 'mental illness' – and of appropriate forms of care. They are often acutely disadvantaged in the health care 'market'.

Once ethnic minority 'consumers' enter the mental health care system, they are likely to receive differential clinical diagnoses. Misdiagnosis resulting from the mislabelling as 'deviant' behaviour or explanations that are entirely normal in certain cultures can determine the type of diagnosis, and thus the treatment 'offered' by a mental health facility (Takeuchi et al. 1999: 554). Also, contrary to the popular assumption that people from culturally diverse backgrounds 'take care of their own' within the extended family, a number of research surveys have shown that carers from these backgrounds are generally unassisted by those outside of their immediate family (e.g. Morse and Messimeri-Kianidis 1997; Plunkett and Quine 1996).

Research undertaken in Australia and internationally into mental health service provision for minority ethnic communities has identified a range of problems experienced by people from such communities, including poverty, racism, social isolation, communication difficulties and the social dislocation associated with migration (e.g. Guarnaccia and Parra 1996; Jayasuriya *et al.* 1992). These problems have been identified in international and national policy as social determinants of mental health. The 'social determinants of health' model – endorsed by the World Health Organization, and reproduced in policy documents at a local level – emphasizes the vital importance of social connectedness, freedom from discrimination and economic participation, for mental health.

In Australia, governments have recently begun to acknowledge, through state and national policy, the need to address at least some of these problems. The National Mental Health Strategy, launched by the Federal Government in 1997, recognizes that people from certain groups, including those from non-English-speaking backgrounds, have particular needs and that these may be variable. Consequently, services should cater for, and be responsive to, the variance both within and between communities (Commonwealth Department of Health and Family Services 1997). The Commonwealth Government has also provided funding of $1 million, over three years, to disseminate information on mental health issues and to conduct research into the needs of people from ethnic minority backgrounds who have been diagnosed with a mental illness. Similarly, in Western Australia, *The Mental Health Plan for Western Australia* (Smith *et al.* 1996) has recognized the need for specific strategies and actions to assist people from non-English-speaking backgrounds who are experiencing 'problems with living'. This plan recognizes that people from such backgrounds should be involved in the planning, delivery and evaluation of mental health services. It also emphasizes the need to train the entire mental health workforce about transcultural issues in service delivery (Smith *et al.* 1996). However, despite these policies and programmes, doubts remain about the ability of services to remain sensitive to differences of culture and language, and of policy-makers (e.g. Commonwealth Department of Health and Aged Care 2000) to develop effective participatory structures, under the rapidly changing conditions of health and welfare.

The very language in which debate about health and welfare is currently couched is of particular concern to those who seek to advance policies that take account of the needs of people from minority and disadvantaged groups. Increasingly, the discourse of rights and entitlements in relation to minority groups has given way to a discourse of the responsibilities and obligations of individual citizens – evident in the concept of 'mutual obligation'. The notion that individuals have a right or a reasonable entitlement to government-protected minimum standards in health, housing, education and social security is displaced increasingly by the idea that individuals have an obligation to make some contribution to the community *as a precondition* for membership of that community (Macintyre 1999). Groups such as the unemployed, sole parents, and even the disabled, are told that in order to receive the support of the community they need to 'give something back in return'. With these changes, it has become more and more difficult to argue that some groups, whether defined by ethnicity, shared language, sexual identity, physical or mental ability, or indeed any criteria, are more deserving of entitlements than others. In the prevailing neo-liberal order, the potential for the erosion of established rights is substantial.

Indeed, many of the rights and entitlements of people from immigrant communities have been effectively withdrawn, or downgraded, through recent federal legislative change. Migrants no longer have the 'right', upon arrival, to support from the Australian social security system, but rather must negotiate an unfamiliar employment market, where vocational qualifications may be unrecognized, and where language difficulties may make it difficult to gain meaningful employment, in the absence of government assistance. In practice, these 'obligations', on the part of recent migrants, appear likely to render the settlement experience even more distressing than in previous years, as the provision of assistance, on the part of the government, has become so conditional as to appear effectively unobtainable.

Nevertheless, Australia, along with other countries who are signatories to United Nations conventions, has certain internationally binding *obligations* under the United Nations' *Principles for the Protection of Persons with Mental Illness and for the Improvement of Mental Health Care*. These state that 'all persons have the right to the best available health care, which shall be part of the health and social care system' and emphasize that people who have been diagnosed with a 'mental illness' should not be discriminated against or disadvantaged. They also assert that each person has a right to be cared for as far as possible in his or her community, and that each person has the right to make meaningful decisions about treatments that are suitable to his or her cultural background (Human Rights and Equal Opportunity Commission 1993).

Exploring the health service user's, particularly the carer's, perspective

In light of these observations, we would argue that an important social justice objective in relation to the mental health care of people from culturally diverse backgrounds is to highlight the experiences of users of mental health services, particularly the unpaid carers of persons suffering mental distress. Thus, in a recent study, we consulted a number of carers from local immigrant communities about their experiences of caring for people diagnosed with mental illness, and their knowledge and views of the accessibility of support services (Kokanovic *et al.* 2001). Participating carers were drawn from the Bosnian, Chinese, Croatian and Polish communities of Perth, Western Australia.

The support services available to carers of people diagnosed with a mental illness were investigated, as were the informal support systems utilized by carers from immigrant communities. Focus group discussions (11) were conducted with members from each of the four communities, and interviews (20) were conducted with health and mental health practitioners who had an interest in, and experience of, cross-cultural health and mental health. Interviews (20) were also conducted with carers from these communities. Issues explored included: carers' understanding of mental health and illness; their 'help-seeking' behaviour; their roles in the lives of their relatives; and their lived experience of the settlement process in Australia.

Perhaps the major feature that differentiates this group of 'consumers' from others engaged in similar caring roles is their common experience of migration, and the effects of this on social integration and well-being. The participants described experiences of social isolation, loneliness, language difficulties and unemployment – or a lack of meaningful employment – as distressing aspects of the settlement experience, which exert a strong influence on 'mental health'. These factors were also described as being relevant to the extent to which carers were aware of, and able to utilize the services available to them. Focus group participants indicated some of the problems faced by newly arrived migrants:

> I think that loneliness is the core of it. When the person is inside four walls they imagine all sorts of things – you remember things that you never thought of because you have so much time on your hands. Time and loneliness ... Migrants very often suffer from isolation. So they're not mentally ill. A lot of people in our community are in danger of nervous breakdown because they are so lonely.
>
> (Polish focus group)

> ... [Problems with living are] linked with having a normal life and all of a sudden coming to a new country with no reason to getting up. Back home they would have had a job and some of the jobs started at 6 am–7 am and running through 3 o'clock/4 o'clock – for them here, the day was too long and nothing to do, nothing to occupy themselves ... All of these [problems] often result in depression ... Urge to work and then not being able to fulfil that because for a variety of reasons. And then of course families with young children, lack of English to support children. ... And losing that is terrible, you know, being a parent, being a successful good parent. Because children were overtaking their roles.
>
> (Croatian focus group)

In describing their encounters with mental health providers, carers reported that they tended to be received with 'culturally appropriate' pamphlets, and referrals, rather than with any immediate and tangible offer of assistance.

> Approaching any organization or any services means that they will give you some pamphlets and 'you can read them, you can go there, approach them'. You go there, and they tell you to go even further. And you walk in a circle, and at the end you decide, that you, on your own, have to take care of it. Isn't it true?
>
> (Polish carer)

Participants from the focus groups were also critical of the tokenistic assistance represented by these brochures. Such comments point to the inadequacy of isolated attempts to remedy the 'information asymmetry' of consumers, in the absence of the provision of any form of 'real help'.

> 'Have you done anything for the ethnic communities?' 'Yes we have, we have so much translated material.' Do I go to someone who I suspect is in serious trouble and say 'Read about it because I think you're in trouble?' No, there is a very great need for a person, a person who will come and not bring papers.
>
> (Polish focus group)

Carers also described the gap between the promises of providers and the reality of the care received. Once 'in the system', it appears, it may be difficult for carers to obtain information about the ongoing care of their family member. Often, it seemed, there was little opportunity for the development of a meaningful relationship between those diagnosed with a mental illness and their carers and providers – and no genuine attempt to encourage the participation of 'consumers'.

Did anyone ever tell you what is happening with your husband?

No, no one, not once. At the beginning the social worker in hospital, who seemed very nice, told me that we will have a lot of talks. But we never did. The social workers are always changing. Sometimes I ring up and get somebody new that I don't know and who knows nothing about my husband's case. I don't know who I'm talking to, and I have to start telling her everything from the beginning. That irritates me. They should have everything on file, and they should know it all, but they don't know anything. My son ... made an appointment with my husband's specialist ... It turned out that there was nothing on file.

(Polish carer)

Some carers also drew attention to the 'mismatch' between the explanations and services 'offered' by mental health service providers and the problems experienced by their charges and their families. The following carer openly queries the diagnosis given to his relative, and offers an alternative explanation of her extreme distress and need for help:

They said it was schizophrenia. But it wasn't schizophrenia. She had a nervous breakdown. She had a lot of pressure in her life. Her children, her husband, the lot. Not so much the children, I think, as the husband. And then she had a nervous breakdown. Particularly not being able to speak English. All of it together ...

(Croatian carer)

Similarly, the following group participant described the experience of an immigrant 'consumer', whose experience and own explanations were dismissed by his GP in favour of a 'cost effective' biological explanation, and a pharmaceutical solution. The complex social account offered by this 'patient' was effectively discounted by the provider:

He went to the doctor and he was trying to explain why he didn't feel very well about going back to school to learn English and why ... why he felt intimidated by all this situation. And that was not relevant for the doctor in the treatment. For the doctor the treatment was just purely medication. So he wasn't referred to any other organizations, and he actually had been discouraged by the doctors to do that, because they said, 'It's just your brain. You need some different doses of chemicals. It has nothing to do with your perception of coming from a different country. You just study too hard.' That sort of approach ...

(Polish focus group)

Service providers often fail to acknowledge alternative explanations for 'disorders' such as schizophrenia and, indeed, the very presence of such accounts may be regarded as a target for 'educational intervention', rather than as a basis for participation on different terms. As a service provider in one of the focus groups explained:

... I've got this case at my centre – the mother knows nothing about mental illness. She has the kind of, you know, traditional thought that schizophrenia is due to spiritual causes, like someone has caused evil things to happen to this person. So therefore they must go and see a medium, someone who can take them out from this evilness or whatever it is. They do not believe in therapy and medication. There are cases like this, where they've carried on in life and they deal with whatever illness they have without help.

And once she was educated she understood it and she allowed her son to take the medication. Because she said, 'Those medications are not helpful. They are doing my son more harm, because they've got side effects.' So, I really think that the Asian community, we should educate people, or carers of mentally ill people. To give them the education and information on what the illness is ...

(Chinese focus group)

Contrary to the rhetoric of consumerism, people diagnosed with mental illness, and their carers, are not always presented with meaningful choices in the health care system. Indeed, consumers of mental health services often lose their right to make such 'choices' on their own behalf. Instead, close relatives – who may or may not be those responsible for daily care and support – are awarded these powers. Unpaid carers who are not close relatives may not be acknowledged in the decision-making process, even when their charge has indicated that, in the event of some incapacity, they would prefer to entrust their carer with this responsibility.

Sometimes I used to think, 'Who can I ring?' When I was really desperate, I couldn't always get the doctor ... And in the end, when things got really bad, I didn't want her to go to [residential psychiatric institution], but that was the only ... sort of alternative. And it was heartbreaking for me, because when she came out of hospital, she said, 'Why did you put me in hospital?' It wasn't our choice; it was her husband's. I felt it wasn't necessary, really. If the right sort of help had been there she would never have had to go to [residential psychiatric institution], because she wasn't one of those cases that had to go, like, to be tied up. And it made her worse.

(Croatian carer)

Carers from immigrant communities are often excluded altogether from discussions about the mental health care of their relative. The exclusion of carers from such discussions seems particularly inappropriate given the centrality of the value of family care in some cultures. The importance of acknowledging and respecting the role of the family in the ongoing support and care of their relatives is underlined by the comments of both focus group participants and mental health practitioners:

They [mental health service providers] don't talk to the family. And how do you expect the carer to be looking after someone if they don't get detailed information? But I think both ways too – there are some doctors who would talk to carers and not the patient.

(Chinese focus group)

In Chinese culture there is no separate self, there is a family self. People are not considered as separate individuals – they are part of the whole family. So when you see a Chinese person you have to realize you have the whole family there. There's no clear boundary between self and family … Sometimes therapy values are not consistent with those of cultural values. Like, 'opening up' is inappropriate in many cultures. Talking about problems does not exist in many cultures … So when you say, 'Talk about your problem,' or, 'Tell me about your problem,' you have already put him or her in conflict because that's not what the culture allows.

(Psychologist)

We have to be very careful because I remember a Greek mother with her son. She said, 'Can you explain to me symbiot. ….What is symbiotic mother? Because the psychiatrist told me that my son is in a symbiotic relationship with me, because he is still living at home. But, in Greek culture, if I have a big house and my son is living in it and if he has an illness, I am his mother and I am taking care of him. It's my obligation to take care of him … And I was told that I'm not letting him go. I'm not letting him individuate.'

(Psychologist)

These accounts give some indication of the role of service providers in contributing to the stigma attached to 'mental illness', and help explain the reluctance of carers and those suffering mental distress from immigrant communities to seek help from mental health practitioners. Culturally inappropriate terminology, questionable diagnoses and treatments that are not consistent with cultural values all contribute to the stigma reportedly accompanying having a mental illness in the family. The secrecy surrounding 'mental illness' and carers' reluctance to seek help outside of the immediate family was explained as being in response to this stigma. A number of carers stressed that stigma often extends to encompass entire families:

Everybody … if they knew you had somebody like that in the family, they would insult you, they looked [sic] at you as though you were different, they looked [sic] at you [as though you] were the same [ie. mentally ill]. If they knew your mother had schizophrenia they thought [sic] everybody in the family had the same problem.

(Croatian carer)

Providing meaningful choices for 'consumers' of mental health care from immigrant communities

Adapting mental health services in order to ensure that 'consumers' from immigrant communities are presented with meaningful choices is unlikely to result from 'top-down' decision-making and change. If changes are to reflect the concerns of service users, mechanisms need to be established for ongoing community participation and consultation. Such sentiments are reflected in various mental health promotion policy documents, both in Australia and internationally. However, a cursory glance at the most recent statistics for consumer participation in Western Australia reveals that only 5 per cent of mental health services have some provision for the inclusion of service users in decision-making, and that these users tend to be from middle-class, English-speaking backgrounds – *not* from ethnic minority immigrant communities (Sozomenou *et al.* 2000). Clearly, more effort needs to be made to engage these 'overlooked' users in the development and evaluation of appropriate mental health services.

The participants in the above study described the kinds of procedural changes that may help to encourage the meaningful participation of carers and consumers from immigrant communities in mental health care. Given the stigma surrounding mental illness, acknowledging and accepting the experiences of people with problems in living was suggested as a crucial step towards addressing the problems of service users from immigrant communities. As one carer explained:

> Acceptance has always been important, looking after them [the mentally ill] and encouraging [them]. By doing so you notice that they get better much quicker. I truly believe that an illness of the mind and thought requires medicines of mind and thought – that is, support and acceptance from family and society. Some mental illnesses require medicines, but more often than not [they] require psychological support. If you give them [the mentally ill] respect and treat them like normal people they will recover very quickly. ... A mental illness is but one type of illness ... they can resume a normal life once they have recovered. But if you do not give them ongoing support it can be very difficult for them. Instead of giving support we often give them bad experiences.
>
> (Chinese carer)

> ... If you put it in terms of simply 'stress' and it's the way a person deals with a very stressful event, rather than some sort of madness that is in them, you change the whole way they approach and look at it and makes it easier for them to deal with. Because it is a huge hurdle for a lot of those people to overcome initially. It's the initial hurdle of 'I need help. I need some assistance with my problem.'
>
> (Counsellor)

It is significant that the form of support requested most frequently by carers was for everyday, practical, material matters – such as help with cleaning, transport and domestic duties. Carers also often indicated that, ultimately, the best form of support for them as carers would be to direct some more meaningful assistance to their relative in need. Other requests included the need for language-specific telephone helplines, and for time out from the daily routines of caring. These suggestions are modest, and clearly do not indicate any desire among carers from immigrant communities to abrogate responsibility for care. Indeed, the requests of carers for further assistance for their relatives points to the interdependence of the needs of those diagnosed with mental illness and their carers in immigrant communities.

Conclusion

As we have argued, the consumer model has limited applicability in health care, and mental health care in particular, in a culturally diverse society. The notion that 'consumers' are sovereign – that is, free of constraint and able to exercise 'informed choice' in 'the market' on the basis of 'perfect' knowledge – is highly questionable in a situation (as exists in most biomedically oriented health care systems) of great inequalities in power and knowledge. Problems with the model are especially apparent where differences in belief and perspective on 'mental illness' and its care, and inequalities in access to resources, undermine assumptions about how people 'normally' think and behave. Further, the absence of information on services, at least in a form that is useful to potential 'consumers'/'clients', and the inability of services to meet needs in a culturally and linguistically sensitive manner, underline the limitations of the consumerism model in relation to the provision of services. Service providers very often do not 'produce' what 'customers' need, or at least not in a form that is experienced as 'user friendly'.

These deficits in mental health service provision are increasingly recognized in national and international policies pertaining to mental health services. However, in the absence of effective participatory structures, it is unlikely that services will be able to produce what immigrant consumers need. Despite mounting evidence of the limitations of the consumer model in health care, consumerism is increasingly manifest in policies in mental health care, in assumptions about people's relationship to professionals and their services, and in the use of language. People are expected to become self-reliant, to be attuned to their own individual health needs, and to participate actively, as 'good' consumers, in the health care market.

In light of the above and the contemporary focus on 'community-based care', it is important to explore the implications of consumerism for those who take the major responsibility for the unpaid care of people described as 'mentally ill'. Some critics have drawn attention to the increasing trend for people to see themselves as health consumers who are prepared, as such, to organize to protect their 'rights'. Since it emerged in the 1980s, the mental health consumer movement has sought to establish control over psychiatric treatment and the stigma accompanying a psychiatric diagnosis, as well as to develop systems of care that cater for the diverse needs and wishes of mental health consumers. Members of the movement have adopted the consumer nomenclature, trading on issues of choice and freedom in an ideal market of mental health services (see Kaufmann 1999: 493–4).

One of the major difficulties encountered by the mental health care consumer movement has been in recruiting members, since people are often reluctant to acknowledge their status as 'mentally ill'. This reluctance is hardly surprising since, as Kaufmann observes, 'mental illness' is unlike most other ways of describing human distress since it calls into question the social worthiness of the person described as 'mentally ill' (1999: 499). Clearly, the movement faces a major challenge in forging a common and positive identity among a diverse population of people who are likely to be physically dispersed and socially isolated. An important goal of movement activists has been to counter the individualization and pathologization of psychological distress and to change the location of 'the problem', from that of the biological-individual to that of the person-in-context. This requires consideration of the social, economic and political determinants of mental health (Kaufmann 1999: 499). One obvious area for action for the mental health consumer movement, as well as for supportive scholars, is to help to shift the frameworks of understanding about mental health care, to make visible people's experiences of the mental health system, and of undertaking unpaid caring work, and to highlight what are often unacknowledged problems faced by 'clients' and their carers in their daily lives. In the same way as activists in the mental health consumer movement have sought to counter the effects of stigma by reframing 'mental illness', there is a need to challenge the assumptions of consumerism in mental health care by reframing perspectives on care. In particular, there is a need to thoroughly interrogate the language in which discussion about care is currently couched.

One practical means to disrupt the terminology used to describe the recipients of mental health services, and to make steps towards their meaningful involvement in decisions about policy, is to appropriate the rhetorical devices of quality and evidence from the consumer-oriented 'evidence-based practice' model. Pilgrim and Rogers (1999) report on a marginal but increasing trend for user-based criterion for 'treatment effectiveness' to be employed in order to unsettle a professional-centred approach to defining the evidence base for mental health service effectiveness. This trend offers one strategy by which the views of users and their carers could be deployed to influence the development of more appropriate mental health services.

A major challenge facing scholars and activists in their efforts to recast the terms of debate about mental health care is that there has developed a politics of consensus surrounding the use of the terms 'community' and 'care'. Although in debate and writing these terms are often left undefined – or are poorly defined – they have strong evaluative connotations, denoting ideals that are embraced by those of diverse political persuasions. Throughout its history, the term 'community' has signified the society of the small-scale, face-to-face interaction and local control. It suggests shared interest and identity and its image stands opposed to that of the society of the large-scale, the remote and impersonal bureaucracy, and professional control (see, e.g., Plant 1974). The term 'care' evokes the ideal of bondedness and self-less devotion to, indeed love of, the other. In the modern Western world, its meanings have been forged in the context of discourse of the nuclear family, with its idealized and romanticized bonds between husband and wife, and parent and child. Few people would argue with the proposition that 'care in the community' (usually meaning care in the family) is generally more humane ('caring') than care in a psychiatric institution. However:

- What does such 'care' mean in practice?
- What role do mental health services play in 'augmenting' such care?
- Who undertakes this caring work?
- What does this work entail?
- What constitutes the 'community' where the caring is presumed to be undertaken?
- What scope is there for marginalized members of 'the community' to voice their concerns and to influence the policies that affect them?

It is evident that there is a need for a thoroughgoing interrogation of the discourse of caring in the context of 'the community'. When considering diverse *communities*, it is important to remain attuned to how an appeal to 'the community' may serve to homogenize differences in backgrounds, viewpoints, opportunities, and needs, and the burdens carried unequally by those (mainly women) who undertake unpaid 'care in the community'. The focus on 'community-based care' potentially entails many benefits for those directly affected and for 'society' as a whole. However, the effect may be to excuse authorities from responsibility for providing the necessary supports for users and their carers, and to divert attention from required changes in economic, political, and social conditions. As consumerism gains pace in mental health care, and health care more generally, the need to acknowledge and value the perspective of those diagnosed with mental illness and their carers – especially those from marginalized culturally diverse groups – is becoming increasingly evident.

Note

1   This chapter draws on some material from a study jointly undertaken by
Renata Kokanovic, Eastern Perth Public and Community Health Unit, and Alan
Petersen, Sociology Programme, Murdoch University, in Western Australia. We
would like to thank everyone who agreed to participate in the study. We are
particularly grateful to Vlasta Mitchell, who assisted with data collection and
analysis. The study was made possible with the financial support offered by the
Eastern Perth Public and Community Health Unit, Perth, Western Australia,
and a Special Research Grant from Murdoch University, Western Australia.

References

Chin, J.L. (2000) 'Culturally competent health care', *Public Health Reports*, 115, 1:
25–33.
Commonwealth Department of Health and Aged Care (2000) *National Action Plan
for Promotion, Prevention and Early Intervention for Mental Health*, Canberra:
Mental Health and Special Programmes Branch, Commonwealth Department of
Health and Aged Care.
Daniel, A. (1998) 'Trust and medical authority', in A. Petersen and C. Waddell (eds)
Health Matters: A Sociology of Illness, Prevention and Care, Sydney: Allen &
Unwin, and London: Sage.
Guarnaccia, P. (1998) 'Multicultural experiences of family caregiving: a study of
African American, European American and Hispanic American families', *New
Directions for Mental Health Services*, 77 (Spring): 45–61.
Guarnaccia, P. and Parra, P. (1996) 'Ethnicity, social status, and families' experiences
of caring for a mentally ill family member', *Community Mental Health Journal*,
32, 3: 243–60.
Hugman, R. (1994) 'Consuming health and welfare', in R. Keat, N. Whiteley and N.
Abercrombie (eds) *The Authority of the Consumer*, London and New York: Rout-
ledge.
Human Rights and Equal Opportunity Commission (1993) *Human Rights and
Mental Illness: Report of the National Inquiry into the Human Rights of People
with Mental Illness*, Vols 1 and 2 (Commissioner Brian Burdekin), Canberra:
Australian Government Printing Service.
Jayasuriya, L., Sang, D. and Fielding, A. (1992) *Ethnicity, Immigration and Mental
Illness: A Critical Review of Australian Research*, Canberra: Australian Govern-
ment Publishing Service.
Kaufmann, C.L. (1999) 'An introduction to the mental health consumer movement',
in A.V. Horwitz and T.L. Scheid (eds) *A Handbook for the Study of Mental
Health: Social Contexts, Theories, and Systems*, Cambridge: Cambridge Univer-
sity Press.
Kokanovic, R., Petersen, A., Mitchell, V. and Hansen, S. (2001) *Care-giving and the
Social Construction of 'Mental Illness' in Immigrant Communities*, Perth: Eastern
Perth Public and Community Health Unit and Murdoch University.
Lefley, H.P. (1999) 'Mental health systems in cross-cultural context', in A.V. Horwitz
and T.L. Scheid (eds) *A Handbook for the Study of Mental Health: Social
Contexts, Theories, and Systems*, Cambridge: Cambridge University Press.

Luntz, J. (1998) 'Why do so few people from non-English speaking backgrounds seek mental health services?', *Migration Action*, 2, 1 (April/May): 1998.

Macintyre, C. (1999) 'From entitlement to obligation in the Australian welfare state', *Australian Journal of Social Issues*, 34, 2: 103–18.

Marmot, M. (1999) *The Social Determinants of Health*, Oxford: Oxford University Press.

Mechanic, D. (1999) 'Mental health and mental illness: definitions and perspectives', in A.V. Horwitz and T.L. Scheid (eds) *A Handbook for the Study of Mental Health: Social Contexts, Theories, and Systems*, Cambridge: Cambridge University Press.

Morse, C. and Messimeri-Kianidis, V. (1997) *Keeping it in the Family: The Health and Social Experiences of Carers in Australian-Greek Families*, Canberra: Department of Immigration and Multicultural Affairs Document and Production Unit.

Mulvaney, J. (1994) 'Medicalization, marginalization and control?', in C. Waddell and A.R. Petersen (eds) *Just Health: Inequality in Illness, Care and Prevention*, Melbourne: Churchill Livingstone.

—— (1998) 'Psychiatric disability and community based care', in A. Petersen and C. Waddell (eds) *Health Matters: A Sociology of Illness, Prevention and Care*, Sydney: Allen & Unwin, and London: Sage.

National Health Strategy (1993) *Help Where Help is Needed*, Issues Paper No. 5, Canberra: National Health Strategy.

National Mental Health Strategy Evaluation Steering Committee, for the Australian Health Ministers Advisory Council (1997) *Evaluation of the National Mental Health Strategy: Final Report*, Canberra: Mental Health Branch, Commonwealth Department of Health and Family Services.

Pilgrim, D. and Hitchman, L. (1999) 'User involvement in mental health service development', in C. Newnes, G. Holmes and C. Dunn (eds) *This is Madness: A Critical Look at Psychiatry and the Future of Mental Health Services*, Herefordshire, UK: PCCS Books, pp. 179–94.

Pilgrim, D. and Rogers, A. (1999) *A Sociology of Mental Health and Illness* (2nd edn), Buckingham: Open University Press.

Plant, R. (1974) *Community and Ideology: An Essay in Applied Social Philosophy*, London: Routledge & Kegan Paul.

Plunkett, A. and Quine, S. (1996) 'Difficulties experienced by carers from non-English speaking backgrounds in using health and other support services', *Australian and New Zealand Journal of Public Health*, 20: 27–32.

Secretary of State for Health (1991) *The Health of the Nation*, London: HMSO.

Shackley, P. and Ryan, M. (1994) 'What is the role of the consumer in health care?', *Journal of Social Policy*, 23: 517–41.

Smith, G., McCavanagh, D., Williams, T. and Lipscombe, P. (1996) *Making a Commitment: The Mental Health Plan for Western Australia*, Perth: The Health Department of Western Australia.

Smith, R. (1997) 'The future of healthcare systems', *British Medical Journal*, 314, 7093: 1495–6.

Sozomenou, A., Mitchell, P., Fitzgerald, M., Malak, A.-E. and Silove, D. (2000) *Mental Health Consumer Participation in a Culturally Diverse Society*, Sydney: Australian Transcultural Mental Health Network.

Takeuchi, D.T., Uehara, E. and Maramba, G. (1999) 'Cultural diversity and mental health treatment', in A.V. Horwitz and T.L. Scheid (eds) *A Handbook for the Study of Mental Health: Social Contexts, Theories, and Systems*, Cambridge: Cambridge University Press.

Chapter 8

The active citizen works hard
Living with chronic heart failure

Margaret Reid and Alexander Clark

Consumerism and health

Among the range of possibilities in which the body can develop, health appears to be a particularly sought end. Acknowledgement that the responsibility for health is attributed to the individual has led to a rethinking of the forces that shape behaviour and an awareness of the processes by which the individual, the body and the self are shaped throughout the life course. Attention to health is given high moral value, as maintaining the healthy body demonstrates a commitment to maintaining one's self-identity. The healthy supple body is viewed not only as a controlled body but one that reflects idealized attitudes in the self (Williams and Bendelow 1998). Changes in the presentation of the body reflect alterations in life experiences as well as being shaped by social and cultural processes. A prominent example of this occurs during chronic illness when the self can be threatened by the resulting loss of control and disruption to identity. Individuals then make considerable effort to maintain their sense of normalcy and continuity by incorporating the meaning of the illness into their sense of self (Bury 1997).

Implicit in the conception of the health consumer is the notion of patient agency, as the individual actively works to maintain and achieve greater self-realization and self-improvement. Understanding the consumer role in this way has a long history as sociologists have demonstrated ways in which consumers of health care are actively involved in the construction of their role (Stimson and Webb 1975; Stacey 1988). Until recently, patient agency was often explored in relation to interactions with health professionals in which the patient, far from simply absorbing the advice and information provided, actively constructs the narrative to present to the health professional and attempts during the consultation to maintain some balance in the relationship (for example, Davis 1988). In this analysis the relationship between patient and health professional undergoes a shift, so that the expert becomes viewed in an advisory role, the patient undertaking more fully the responsibility for shaping the management of his or her condition.

The concept of the idealized healthy body is linked to consumer culture.

Working to maintain health is implicit in everyday discourses, the trim body being maintained through energetic consumption of certain foods, particular forms of activity and a lifestyle in which health maintenance is paramount. On the other hand, poor health itself is seen as 'distasteful' (Lupton 1995), and a lack of fitness, poor body tone and an ageing body suggests a falling away of control and a lack of attention to the lifelong project. Chronic illness, the focus of this chapter, presents particular problems for those attempting to achieve this ideal. The maintenance of a healthy body cannot always be sustained and chronic illness makes the above ideal appear unachievable. Nevertheless, the project is not abandoned; medication and self-management combine in the struggle to maintain health and normality. Continued attempts are demanded to carry out those activities that appear to allow a 'healthy' life, and the constant vigilance of fluctuating boundaries around an uncertain life requires work. Using the condition of heart failure as illustrative, the chapter utilizes the concepts of struggle and work to examine the issues around the active consumer failing to maintain a healthy body.

In a self-conscious analysis to demonstrate the demanding nature of this form of activity, Corbin and Strauss (1988) focus upon the work of the chronic patient. However, their conceptualization of 'work' was very task-oriented, using examples of taking medication as illness-related work and housekeeping as everyday work. The notion that being sick is *hard work* has been developed in more recent studies of the chronically ill (Williams 1996). In this chapter we would wish to take the argument further, demonstrating (as have others, such as Bury (1982) and Williams (1996)) that work is a symbolic as well as a practical activity. The chronically ill are therefore practising health consumerism, although the outcome may not be health, but regulated or managed ill-health.

Research in the field of chronic illness and disability has already extended the realm of interest from patients to the 'sufferers' of chronic illness (Radley 1994). To understand how the sufferer manages his or her condition necessitates entering the perspective of the chronically ill and studying how they cope with the diagnosis and the demands made by the condition on their lives. This perspective has resulted in research which describes the incorporation of the condition into daily lives and identifies the reconstruction of the self as a sufferer (Williams 2000). Much of the chronic disease literature focuses upon this process, i.e. on the 'biographical disruption' caused by the diagnosis (Bury 1982) and the diminished definition of self which emerges as the condition progresses (Charmaz 1983). This reconstruction and management work will be carried out away from dialogue with members of the medical profession who participate only in certain situations as influential figures in the development of self (Kelly and Field 1998).

Although heart failure is a common chronic condition, relatively little is known about its management in a day-to-day sense or the impact of the condition on the individual's self and identity. The broader biomedical literature is primarily concerned with the topic of compliance (Donovan 1995), thus representing a paternalistic model of decision-making about medication which fails to acknowledge the extensive work which individuals carry out in relation to this task. In terms of heart failure, the compliance literature is extensive, fostered by the argument that non-compliance leads to expensive re-hospitalization (Ghali et al. 1988). The notion that men and women with heart failure take an active and 'expert' approach to its management contravenes much of this existing literature which has emphasized instead the passivity of the 'patient' and the lack of commitment to medication-taking. The moral status of patients is judged by their ability to conform to professional prescriptions; thus 'good' patients are those who comply, and non-compliers are viewed as failures (Thorne 1990).

Our chapter aims to demonstrate that individuals with heart failure work at becoming expert in the management of their condition. We concentrate upon two central areas of management, the first being medication work, the second, monitoring of the body. Donovan argues for, and this chapter provides an example of, a 'sufferer-oriented' understanding of medication-taking in which individuals acknowledge the difficulties of routine medication work but attempt ways of incorporating medication-taking into their daily routines. Part of this work is concerned with normalizing medication-taking so that the individual is able to sustain a healthy body approach.

As we have noted, being fit and active has a high cultural value, and yet for individuals with chronic heart failure, commitment to the healthy body project becomes decreasingly likely as their currency, measured in terms of energy, diminishes and the body becomes liable to sudden 'breakdown'. The chapter begins by examining medication work, while the second part focuses upon strategies of health maintenance, establishing a self-surveillance system to monitor the body cues at all times in order to minimize exposure to risk. Most remain actively engaged in constructing their lives in a meaningful way, becoming expert at assessing and avoiding risk, and attempting to maintain independent lives. Nevertheless, they are aware of the ways in which the boundaries shrink and the choices and life opportunities open to them become less and less available.

Heart failure

Heart failure is a clinical condition characterized by shortness of breath, oedema (or fluid retention) and fatigue or poor exercise tolerance (US Department of Health 1994). It is a chronic condition, brought on by left ventricular dysfunction. Recent improvement in the management of heart failure through a new generation of drugs has modified the symptoms and extended the life expectancy of those suffering from the condition. Thus individuals with heart failure cannot recover their health, but can attempt to maintain some kind of stability with the condition although the outcome is always mortality. Life expectancy in Scotland after diagnosis is on average two years (McIntyre *et al.* 2000).

Our data are derived from a study of men and women with chronic heart failure and their carers, living in the west of Scotland. A sample of 50 men and women (36 and 14 respectively) and 30 carers were interviewed in their home by one of us (AC). The interviews focused on patients' and carers' knowledge of heart failure, its impact on their lives, their approach to its management and their interactions with health professionals. Interviews lasted between 50 minutes and 3 hours.

The interviews were transcribed and analysed using key themes identified inductively with the help of NUD: IST, a computer program that assists with the management and analysis of qualitative data. The individuals were sampled from one outpatient clinic in a local hospital. Inclusion criteria for the study are important to acknowledge, as they affect the representation of heart failure reported below. We sampled only those under 80 years of age with a diagnosis of heart failure; individuals interviewed were diagnosed as having New York Heart Association (NYHA) type II and III heart failure – that is, mild to moderate heart failure, individuals being symptomatic but not critically ill.

Medication work: setting up the routines

Individuals with heart failure had to work hard to achieve some form of stability in their lives. Medication was seen to contribute to that stability and the importance of medication-taking was stressed from the time of diagnosis. All participants reported that they saw taking regular medication as important. Reasons for this determination differed, with some individuals citing the necessity of following their doctor's advice (regardless of any perceived benefit), while others linked the medication-taking directly to the preservation of health. Failure to do so carried the potential of a 'crisis' with the individual experiencing increased fluid retention, breathing problems, and ultimately emergency hospitalization. Thus the establishment of the routine helped to ensure attention to the body project, contributing to the maintenance of good health and, second, the avoidance of risk.

Setting up and maintaining the routines was not straightforward. As heart failure is more common in the elderly and those with existing heart-related problems (such as a previous heart attack or high blood pressure) individuals with heart failure often take many other medications associated with chronic or cardiac-related conditions, all of which have their own requirements regarding frequency. In this study the number of tablets individuals were prescribed ranged from 5 to 20 per day, with an average of 10, with participants often taking the medication at several different times of day. Creating order and routine out of such a complex regimen involved considerable planning, as Mr Yorke explains (all respondents have been given pseudonyms):

MR YORKE: No, I try to regulate it. I take one of the enalapril [ACE inhibitor] in the morning, perhaps around eight o'clock in the morning, and the two frusamide [diuretic] in the morning, and the digoxin in the morning because they are all prescribed in the morning. And [I] leave the final enalapril to eight o'clock at night or thereabouts. Which evens out the medication to the body.

Some used commercially produced boxes (which separated out doses into times of day and days of the week), others constructed their own *aide memoires* that resembled the commercial devices but were tailored to the individual's present regimen and preferences in their design, size and number of compartments.

AC: Have you always organized the tablets in that way with the wee box?
MR JOHNSON: No, just when I came into the big doses. I did my best, [I was] going like that 'One, two' ... [as if counting out the tablets individually]. I fix them on a Saturday now and when it comes to Sunday I just fill them all up again. Eleven tablets in each box ...

AC: Have you always organized them that way with the box?
MR BRIDGES: It's the only way to remember, believe it or not ... Before I did [it this way], my tablets were in the bag that the chemist gave me them. They would be lying at the side of the chair and my wife would say, 'Would you not tidy them?' Anyway, I would put them away in a cupboard and forget to take them because they weren't there. But this thing [home made box] goes with me everywhere I go.

Individuals reported a range of strategies that they had developed to minimize medication work. For many of the sample, taking tablets had become an established item of work that was incorporated into their day. For some, the intention was to create a routine so perfect that they were unaware of its intrusion into their lives, thus living 'healthy' lives that were facilitated by medication.

MR GEORGE: No, it gets to the point where it's something that you have got to do. If you like, it's a chore. There are nine pills I take in a day. It's eight in the one [section of the box], and one later on. It tends to be, you get fed up looking at them, 'Not this again', you stand swallowing them all back. But that is about as much as really goes through your head with them. It's pills I have been told to take so I take them.

MR MCALPINE: I deal with myself automatically more or less. I know when they are due and when I am supposed to take them, so I just carry on that way.

As heart failure progresses, the medication individuals are prescribed changes in terms of type and dosage. This results in established regimes becoming subject to periodic change. Individuals reported that, in these circumstances, a pattern of medication-taking had to be (re)constructed, the routine becoming less implicit and the task requiring relearning. In the following quotation, Mrs Saunders describes teaching Mr Saunders again about his drugs:

MRS SAUNDERS: [Mr Saunders has heart failure.] I do [organize] the tablets, we get the pills [from the chemist] and I get them out and I show him. 'Right we start with morning ones', I said: 'Forget about names, there is the boxes and the boxes tell you that it is your morning ones.' So we do the boxes, that is 'a.m.' and I said 'Right, lunch time is your three water [tablets]. That is another box there.' So I am trying to teach him like that, he is doing not bad. He is coming on. He has got to learn because there could be a time, I could be away, at our age.

MR BRIDGES: The wife, she'll say to me every night in life, 'Have you taken your tablet?' Even if she goes out [which she doesn't often] she might go out and she'll come back and say, 'Did you remember and take your tablets?' And I'll say 'I did'.

Interviewees who lived with a carer (partner) frequently discussed medication-taking as a shared activity, the carer and the heart failure individual taking equal responsibility. These two quotations indicate that the respondent and carer become co-workers on the body project. The active consumer discourse assumes that the individual acts autonomously and that while strategies may be developed in consultation with others, the responsibility for the project is shouldered alone. This study provides examples of a shared discourse, where both the sufferer and the carer work jointly to try to maintain the health of the individual.

Medication and risk

For those with heart failure, constant medication-taking is a basic requirement to sustain a 'normal' life. Medication-taking is, we have demonstrated, complex, given the range and variation in the timing and quantity of the different drugs; it was also risky work. One of the main risks was running low, or out of drugs. The biomedical literature reported patients taking 'drug holidays' (Fawcett 1995). Our respondents argued strongly that they were highly committed to setting up and maintaining these regimes, but also reported times when they ran low on drugs or simply forgot to take them. Failure to take the drugs could trigger a crisis, and knowledge of this possibility resulted in people reporting great caution regarding maintaining their drug supply:

MRS HIGGINS: [who cares for Mr Higgins] I always like to have enough that when I see it [number of tablets in box] going down I know, 'Oh this won't last over the weekend' and put in for a prescription and get it that day. Then I know then that he is covered for the week until it goes down.

Strategies for monitoring the supply include sharing the responsibility with the carer, as did Mr Higgins, but also finding allies to help to avert the crisis. A friendly pharmacist was cited as one such person. Mrs Chalmers is typical when she answers the question of how many times she/they had been without tablets: 'Never, because the chemist will just give us them in advance and he takes them back when we hand in the prescription.'

The risk of running low or out of drugs demonstrates the fragility of the respondents as 'healthy' people. Such a risk creates a constant tension between establishing the routine that allows medication-taking to be taken for granted and, on the other hand, maintaining a sufficient self-awareness to ensure that the medication has actually been taken. Some respondents commented on the anxiety surrounding the difficulty in remembering that the medications had been taken:

MRS NEIL: [reports on her internal dialogue on the issue] Oh God, I went into the room to take them, I wonder if I took them, you know what I mean? And I says to myself, I'm sure I took them, no I didn't, but then again I say to myself, I can't have taken them ...

Monitoring the body

We have argued that medication-taking is central to the role of the heart failure sufferer as active citizen. Individuals respond to the necessity of medication by creating routines that minimize the work, thereby reducing the constant reminder of ill-health; in turn the medication helps sustain a reasonable state of 'health'. However, certain forms of action (for example, overactivity) carried the risk of bringing on breathlessness and fluid build-up in their lungs, and the possibility of emergency hospitalization. Thus their work as moral citizens required them to be ever vigilant and the habit of monitoring their bodily state became a further task under the rubric of 'health work'. If monitoring was well accomplished then the healthy body project continued to be successful. If unsuccessful, then an unhealthy body state became quickly apparent; and remedial action was required. This could be through *in*-activity, or through changing the drug regimen. Either way, the sufferers had to work hard to try to re-establish a 'healthy' life.

The lay understanding of the body has become a significant topic of interest within the field of chronic illness, with researchers of chronic diabetes leading the way in the literature on 'reading bodily cues' (Hernandez *et al.* 1999; Paterson and Sloan 1994). In diabetes, lack of blood sugar creates an imbalance in the system which has to be remedied through the taking of insulin; signs of an insulin crisis become familiar to the individual who acts quickly to change the imbalance. For individuals with heart failure, we will argue, reading cues is a central aspect of body monitoring. In this case, the monitored currency is energy expenditure, with imbalances being created when energy reserves are over-stretched. In such situations, the body was seen as being unable to carry out even basic routines (respondents described the difficulties of washing up a tea cup and saucer) and the identity of themselves as chronically ill became dominant.

To guard against this many of our interviewees reported that they learned to monitor their body, listening to the physical cues ('Oh, I've got a sort of bloaty feeling today' Mrs Fay) and responding if necessary. Self-monitoring was embedded into their everyday lives but unlike the establishment of medication-taking where individuals tried to incorporate the task into their daily routines to the point where the activity became taken for granted, body-monitoring is referred to as a self-conscious task.

MR MCALPINE: If I go down to [place] to see all the boys and they are all in a conversation and laughing. If I talk too long you can actually hear it [voice] fading away because I have used up too much energy, there is nothing there ... It's when you relax again, the body seems to say 'Right, that is you built up again'.

MR GEORGE: You pace yourself, you take your time now, well I do. Your body tells you at some point you have done enough, it's time to sit down and as soon as I feel this and it's just a feeling ... I just get the feeling, that's it, you're done.

AC: You feel it in your body?

MR GEORGE: You feel it in your body, that's it, but it's very very hard, I can't put it into words. But it's just as if your body is telling you 'Right that's it, it's time to sit down'. How can I put it? I can't put it into words, it's like that tiredness when it comes over you. It's like somebody just drawing a silk sheet over your face, one minute you are sitting there and then whoosh.

Self-monitoring is part of everyday health work, present in the self-surveying activities of individuals as they judge themselves against others. In circumstances where a missed cue could lead to a critical health problem, however, such activity assumes a particular importance. Individuals become expert in the ways in which the condition may affect their own body and develop what Hernandez calls the 'science of one'. By this is meant respondents go beyond medical signs and symptoms to prioritize particular bodily sensations which they feel are of importance to them (Hernandez *et al.* 1999).

Characteristic of self-monitoring is the internal dialogue which many report, a discussion between the body and the 'sensible' self.

MR GEORGE: Yes, there are certain things, and if it comes to you to want to move the furniture around the sitting room, you need to say 'Wait a minute, rule me out of that one. I am not going to attempt that.' There are things that you will say: 'Right I won't do that.' It is mainly, carrying things, you are limited to what you can carry and the distance that you can go.

MRS JENKINS: Then I find that I am terribly breathless and my chest gets tighter and tighter and I think 'Wait a minute, I have done enough' and I have to stop. You just get to know.

As with medication work, *self*-monitoring was often shared work. Although usually referred to as *self*-monitoring – an activity carried out by the individual – monitoring work can be shared between a couple. In the study, many examples emerged of co-monitoring, most often with the two partners sharing in monitoring the individual with heart failure, but very occasionally, explicit co-monitoring occurred when each attended to themselves as well as the other. Co-monitoring involved not only a shared knowledge of signs and symptoms but also, for the partner, an ability to read the body of the sufferer.

The currency of energy

Nowhere is the pressure on individuals to be physically active citizens more clearly evident than with those who find it difficult to do so. Physical activity is highly valued in our society and viewed as being righteous, and by the same token, inactivity is not. 'Who wants to lie around?' asked Mr McAlpine. Inactive individuals were perceived negatively by many respondents, and while a few recognized that their active lives were largely past, many worked hard to sustain a conception of themselves as still achieving some measure of their former lives and the domestic and social roles they associated with it.

The central currency with heart failure sufferers was energy. Energy could be hoarded, saved, spent and re-collected. The 'new' energy-conserving way of life often contrasted with the former life in which energy was not hoarded in the same manner. Indeed descriptions of life before 'the turning point' often appeared to exaggerate the carefree way in which activities were carried out.

AC: Would it be fair to say that you take quite a paced approach?
MR KING: Oh I don't run about like a twenty-year-old, those days have gone by.

The recognition that many forms of activity were now literally and metaphorically out of bounds was difficult for those individuals whose previous employment assumed a certain level of physical fitness – in our interviews most notably those who had worked in skilled or semi-skilled manual employment. Thus a number of men (though fewer women) made reference to their former abilities and the new circumscribed life:

MR BRIGGS: Oh it slows you down something terrible. There are no climbing ladders, no climbing stairs or anything like that now. I was a crane driver in the shipyards and you have about 60 foot to climb [to get into the crane]. That is you going up. That was taboo that. Just brought on an angina attack all the time.

AC: What kinds of things, other things, would you tend not to do now that you did before?
MR JONES: Well doing anything heavy. Light things I can do, like make cups of tea, or anything like that. If I was to lift only a heavy box, I could take it up the stairs no bother. But now I leave it at the bottom and I say to my wife, 'I can't lift it.' I hesitate, I am frightened of bringing this [breathlessness] on again.

Boundary maintenance

Monitoring the body was carried out by first establishing boundaries that would allow our respondents to carry on living without setting the body at excessive risk. Boundaries are symbolic, described by the individuals in terms of what he or she perceived as being possible in their lives, and what lay beyond that, unachievable. Thus heart failure sufferers reported having to establish an understanding of what tasks could be undertaken or roles fulfilled on a specific day or during a specific stage of the heart failure. Wiener talks of the forces of pain and disability shaping the lives of those with rheumatoid arthritis, documenting how sufferers learn to monitor their body for readings of these components of their life (Wiener 1975). In the case of those with heart failure the shaping force was (a lack of) energy, and it was this energy 'reading' which set the boundaries of their social world.

Boundaries were influenced by significant others, including the partner, medical opinion and broader social conceptions about the condition. They could be expressed in a number of ways, most literally as geographical boundaries, as men and women described physical destinations beyond their reach (for example, towns and cities a distance away), and climatic, since being physically active in certain weathers was more difficult (windy weather). Boundaries could be expressed as social, in terms of the limits to the kind of social occasions which they would not attend – usually those that were seen as being too demanding (for example, involving a large family gathering or group of friends).

Critically, other boundaries were set around physical activities in which they could no longer engage, such as active sports, walking (especially uphill) and many forms of manual activities such as gardening and do-it-yourself around the house. Heart failure patients (especially those within the categories of our study) may experience months (or even years) of reasonable stability. Despite this, boundaries required constant monitoring and this very self-conscious activity established itself as central to their lives. Some developed recipes to support their attitude to living, such as Mrs Royce whose motto was 'Don't rush', Mr Rankin's was 'Be sensible' while Mr Andrews' was 'Take your time'. These and others represented ways in which individuals justified their slower, energy-saving approach to life. Creating new boundaries from the taken-for-granted ones was not necessarily an easy task. Interviewees reported making mistakes, trying out former activities which overtaxed them, while the partner had also to learn the boundaries of his or her spouse. In one instance, there was some conflict until the partner, Mrs Briggs, realized that new boundaries had been set.

MRS BRIGGS: I could have done with help how to cope with it, I don't know. I just felt 'He is there, he is fine, he looks fine so he should be able to do it'. And it wasn't. I would moan at him for sitting about: 'Why are you sitting about? Why aren't you up trying to do this? Come on, you have to go to … ' You know, I had no idea, I was really hopeless.

AC: So you felt almost as if you wanted to do more?

MRS BRIGGS: No, I felt as if I wanted him to do more.

It has been argued that moral citizenship involves a commitment to being physically active, to walking, playing games, and to being engaged with a range of projects that demonstrate an awareness and commitment to fitness and health. With the ageing and ill, such commitments become difficult. One way for those with chronic heart failure to retain such commitment was by reducing physical activity to a lower achievable level to minimize the risk of over-stepping the boundary.

MR JONES: Even going for my paper, I can't do that now, I hesitate doing that.

AC: Is that up the road?

MR JONES: Yeah, in case I take a bad turn. I got a fright that last time when I reached the car. I knew I wasn't going to make it so I just came back.

This low-risk approach involved attempting only tasks and activities that were tried and tested. Unfamiliar situations such as a relative's wedding, or one in which the end point could not be guaranteed (for example, tackling a task in the home which could uncover further problems) created uncertainty, and fear and anxiety were counter-posed with the security of the familiar. Terminology emphasized protection, safeness, not taking chances; for example, 'I'm safeguarding myself.'

While many taking the low-risk approach would continue to carry out a number of tasks, a few reported feeling so anxious that they had virtually stopped most forms of activity. Of all our 'active citizens', these 'non-risk' citizens who experienced this anxiety were the least active and had the more developed stage of heart failure [NYHA type III].

MR COOK: I'm too afraid to do any more. At one time I used to walk to the paper shop in the morning, I used to get the pains in the chest, I would stop and use the spray. I believe it's the cold air, you know, the cold air.

On the other hand, one or two individuals (in our small sample, more women than men) quite consciously took a high-risk approach, challenging the boundaries, acknowledging the danger involved in doing so. For Mr Jones the choice of exceeding his energies was deliberate, reflecting a desire to 'pass' as a regular grandfather playing with his grandson, with the knowledge that he would pay for such an action at a later date.

MR JONES: There was one occasion recently when my grandson came over and he wanted to go to the park and after a while he wanted to go down and walk along the riverside. He moves very fast, and I carried on and by the time I got halfway through this, it must have been nearly a mile, I was almost on my hands and knees. I was like a drunk man staggering from side to side because I was feeling so weak. And eventually I got through most of it, stopping often on the way to try to compose myself.

Mrs Allison reported deliberately testing the limits of her physical activity by trying, and failing, different sporting activities.

MRS ALLISON: I tried aerobics but that was disaster, that was a nightmare. I came out and the girl who was taking the class came out and said 'Are you finding the exercises difficult?' 'Just a bit' I said, 'I've got heart failure.' 'Just take things easy then' [she said] and I said 'No, I think I will come out.' So I came out and went into the pool and just did a bit of swimming because then I can pace myself and do my own thing. I tried that line dancing, that was another disaster, that was terrible.

In both instances the capacity to be physically active [to engage in the healthy body project] was unrealistic and served to underline both the pressure, even with severe chronic illness, to try to attain this goal and also their inability to honour their commitment.

Overstepping boundaries also occurred, less dramatically, when the condition simply worsened and individuals found that they were not capable of carrying out former activities. On these occasions there was more active work on boundary re-creation, this time in a smaller, diminished world in which the person lived as a decreasingly well-rounded individual.

For this group of respondents, energy expenditure was measured with increasing precision. As opposed to helping to wash up after a meal, or doing housework, they could undertake washing but not drying the cups, smoothing but not making the bed; these were the reduced activities for the individuals who were at a more serious stage of heart failure. The choice of being an active consumer diminishes as there are fewer areas of consumption to engage with, only the possession of a car protecting the individual for a while by allowing greater mobility and more life opportunities.

Discussion

Active citizenship implies a commitment to health and the body project. In this case, those with heart failure and their carers engaged in continuous self-surveillance of the body, focusing upon two key areas, medication-taking and body-monitoring, as central to their attempts at the maintenance of health. Previous perspectives have viewed those with heart failure as approaching medication-taking casually, essentially placing low priority on the task. Instead we have argued that the complexities of the medication require individuals to work hard at establishing and maintaining the routine, which on changing the medication, may require re-evaluating.

While it is the case that our respondents listened to medical advice, they were not passive in their acceptance of the biomedical approach, but adapted professional discourses relating to illness management and incorporated lay discourses to meet their own needs for an active life. Only by drawing upon a broader range of sources (lay and professional) could the illness be managed and attempts at the ideal, 'healthy' self prove successful. Furthermore, both those with heart failure and carers become highly attuned to subtle fluctuations caused by the failing heart to the body. Control and regulation of the body was exercised through the monitoring of energy and the drawing of boundaries associated with roles and activities. These ensured that bodies were not placed at excessive risk while individuals tried to maintain a regulated form of sickness. Overriding, however, was the moral imperative of being active in the face of an incurable illness.

Finally we have made the point that while commitment to the healthy body is often presented as a solitary discourse, this is not necessarily always the case. Co-working was evident in many of the couples that we interviewed, when the single project became a shared one. The concept of the shared project has been little explored in the literature on chronic illness, yet, for many sufferers, working to achieve normality is a shared task, discussed and implemented by the sufferer and his or her partner. In these instances the active citizen becomes plural, and the working together becomes joint labour.

Acknowledgements

We should like to thank the patients and the carers who participated so willingly in this study, our co-grant holders (David Murdoch, John McMurray, Caroline Morrison and Simon Capewell), who have contributed to the development of the ideas in this chapter, and the Scottish Executive, Chief Scientist Office, for funding this study.

References

Bury, M. (1982) 'Chronic illness as biographical disruption', *Sociology of Health and Illness*, 4: 2: 167–82.
—— (1997) *Health and Illness in a Changing Society*, London: Routledge.
Charmaz, K. (1983) 'Loss of self: a fundamental form of suffering in the chronically ill', *Sociology of Health and Illness*, 5: 168–95.
Corbin, J.M. and Strauss, A. (1988) *Unending Work and Care: Managing Chronic Illness at Home*, London: Jossey-Bass.
Davis, K. (1988) *Power Under the Microscope*, Amsterdam: Foris Publications.
Donovan, J.L. (1995) 'Patient decision making: the missing ingredient in compliance research', *International Journal of Technology Assessment in Health Care*, 11, 3: 443–55.
Fawcett, J. (1995) 'Compliance: definitions and key issues', *Journal of Clinical Psychiatry*, 56 (supp. 1): 4–10.
Ghali, J.K., Kadakia, S., Cooper, R. and Ferlinz, J. (1988) 'Precipitating factors leading to decompensation of heart failure', *Archives of Internal Medicine*, 148: 2113–16.
Hernandez, C.A., Bradish, G.I., Rodger, N.W. and Rybansky, S.I. (1999) 'Self-awareness in diabetes: using body cues, circumstances, and strategies', *Diabetes Educator*, 25, 4: 576–84.
Kelly, M. and Field, D. (1998) 'Conceptualising chronic illness', in D. Field and S. Taylor (eds) *Sociological Perspectives on Health, Illness and Health Care*, Oxford: Blackwell.
Lupton, D. (1999) *Risk*, London: Sage.

McIntyre, K., Capewell, S., Stewart, S., Chalmers, J.W.T., Boyd, J., Finlayson, A. *et al.* (2000) 'Evidence of improving prognosis in heart failure: trends in case fatality in 66,547 patients hospitalized between 1986 and 1995', *Circulation*, 102: 1126–31.

Paterson, B.L. and Sloan, J. (1994) 'A phenomenological study of the decision-making experience of individuals with long-standing diabetes', *Canadian Journal of Diabetes Care*, 18, 4: 10–19.

Radley, A. (1994) *Making Sense of Illness: The Social Psychology of Health and Disease*, London: Sage.

Stacey, M. (1988) *The Sociology of Health and Healing*, London: Unwin Hyman.

Stimson, G. and Webb, B. (1975) *Going to See the Doctor: The Consultation Process in General Practice*, London and Boston: Routledge & Kegan Paul.

Thorne, S.E. (1990) 'Constructive noncompliance in chronic illness', *Holistic Nursing Practice*, 5, 1: 62–9.

US Department of Health (1994) *Heart Failure: Evaluation and Care of Patients with Left-Ventricular Systolic Dysfunction*, Maryland: US Department of Health and Human Services.

Wiener, C.L. (1975) 'The burden of rheumatoid arthritis: tolerating the uncertainty', *Social Science and Medicine*, 9: 97–104.

Williams, S.J. (1996) 'The vicissitudes of embodiment across the chronic illness trajectory', *Body and Society*, 2, 2: 23–47.

—— (2000) 'Chronic illness as biographical disruption or biographical disruption as chronic illness?: Reflections on a core concept', *Sociology of Health and Illness*, 22, 1: 40–67.

Williams, S.J. and Bendelow, G. (1998) *The Lived Body: Sociological Themes, Embodied Issues*, London: Routledge.

Chapter 9

The commodification of health in sexually transmitted infections (STI) clinics

Anthony Pryce

Introduction

There are few sites more illustrative of the reconfiguring of the patient as client/consumer and the professional as purveyor of health service commodity, than the sexually transmitted infections (STI) clinic. This chapter is partly an account of the relationship between medicine and sexualities, but is primarily concerned with the consumption by male clients of increasingly commodified sexual health services. It will explore that transaction and draws on data from the 'Eros Project', a study of two sexual health clinics in the UK.

The clients are consumers of two competing and often incompatible rationalities – erotic desire on the one hand and neo-liberal biomedical orthodoxies on the other. Despite the apparent changes in contemporary social and professional attitudes and values, the clinic is an arena where clients confess and catalogue their sexual behaviours. There is also a consistent drive for the client to adopt normalizing health promotion beliefs. Knowing that there will be a pressure 'to tell' will mean that, for some clients, the decision to attend the clinic may require elaborate discretion management. However, some other men integrate clinic attendance into an *informed* sexual lifestyle where the individual is engaged in monitoring the self. This constant self-surveillance for signs of ill health, potential disease and the maintenance of *healthy* regimes is a characteristic of what Armstrong (1995) termed the 'active patient'.

This notion of the 'active patient' developed from Foucault's analyses of 'governmentality' (Lupton 1995), and it is an important aspect in the processes of health consumption, which Turner (1984) has outlined. Foucault (1991) argued that governmentality developed in the eighteenth century as a mechanism for regulating and controlling populations through an apparatus of increasing complexity. Governmentality operates through forms of knowledge(s) (*savoirs*) and institutions such as the law, religion and medicine that exercise moral authority and are coercive influences on society and the individual. These institutions or systems are also normative, and exert power through disciplinary knowledge and practices (such as medicine or psychiatry) on populations and individuals who internalize these as 'ways of seeing'. Drawing on the design for a 'model' prison called the Panopticon (all seeing) designed by Jeremy Bentham in the eighteenth century, Foucault describes how this provides the basis whereby individuals and populations can be governed through the simple device of regulating themselves through self-monitoring in everyday life. One example of governmentality, explored by Nettleton (1995), is how mothers are recruited through dentistry to deploy correct techniques of tooth-brushing and instil regimes of dental hygiene in their children. Similarly, the STI clinic provides another good illustration of medical power being deployed through the panoptic gaze of the clinic. Thus, even in their everyday lives clients are recruited into the regime of self-monitoring for signs of disease and apparently regulating their sexual behaviours to comply with sexual health directives such as 'safer sex'.

However, in relation to sexual health as self-monitoring citizens or 'active patients', men's strategic consumption of the clinic services reveal that they are not just passive, docile consumers. Several tactics that men use in the clinical interaction form a resistance to the medical practices. This resistance may include how much information the client might reveal to doctors and nurses, and whether they tell accurate histories of their sexual activities. The client may not comply with a treatment regime. Even though the client might suspect or know that he has an infection, he might not attend the clinic at all. Whether or not a person chooses to enter the clinical system is a complex process. The process of the individual becoming a consumer of health services raises a number of central issues that are foregrounded here and explored in this chapter.

The first issue stems from the question: What are these clinics and who are the patients that attend? The STI clinic provides a good example of Armstrong's (1995) model of the dispensary as a site of surveillance of populations. This draws on Foucault's analysis of the disciplinary gaze of medicine extending from the examination of the patient in the clinic to the community outside the clinic walls. Much of the data collected from clients by STI clinics are concerned with the mapping of the interpersonal connections of *cases* of infection. However, clinics are also engaged with the commodification of sexual health through their ideologies and practices in the wider context of political and social anxieties around sexual behaviours and risk. They are concerned with advising, educating and the (often) interdisciplinary researching of sexual health that tend to require the client to occupy specific roles as a sexual identity, such as 'gay', 'straight' or bisexual. Clearly, that means that the client must take decisions on whether or not confession of their sexual desires, social roles and sexual praxis will conform to the medico-social models of sexuality and sexual health. This is a key, implicit element in the process of consumption of services by clients and consumption of the production and reproduction of scientific sexual ideologies by staff.

The second key issue is how the examination, identification and treatment of lesions to the genital and elimination systems of the consumer's body are managed. This reflects wider social tensions in terms of both professional–lay interaction and the epistemology of the sexual body, not least, as medically and socially there is an element of the *untouchable* in the nature of sexual diseases. The development of modern medicine has tended to separate the part of the body under examination from the rest of the body. Thus, the sign of disease, such as a genital wart for example, is charted with no reference to the individual or social meanings surrounding the infection and the erotic circumstances of how it was acquired. This focus on the purely behavioural and empirical basis of disease works to reduce the challenge of those meanings that might destabilize conventional social assumptions of sexual categories or identities. For example, a married man who might normally identify as heterosexual, yet secretly maintains 'deviant' sexual desires and activities with women or other men, will have to make decisions about the information he confesses in terms of discretion management in his consumption of clinic services.

Finally, the third issue concerns the consumer's experience of the clinic and how the clinic lays claim to privileged forms of expert knowledge. Some of those who attend the clinic might not feel 'ill', or indeed have symptoms of disease. They often tend to be well, active, people (though potentially discredited through having an STI and attending a clinic!) who have been consumers of erotic desire and practices. At the heart of these issues, of course, is the need to access health care services by 'clients' who make tactical, consumerist decisions about attending the clinic. These clients often need to employ sophisticated strategies for the management of self within the clinical encounter, where the consumption of desire is the subject of both medicalized and erotic discourses.

These three issues were at the heart of the study that will now be described. However, it is important to consider briefly how the research was undertaken and then explore processes whereby the individual client becomes a consumer and the clinic deals in sexual health as a commodity.

The Eros study

The description of the process of consumerization of clients and the commodification of the clinic is drawn from data gathered during the Eros study (Pryce 2000a; 2000b). The aim of that research was to explore the encounter between forms of social and professional knowledge(s), through an exploration of the experience of patients who attend an STI clinic and the professional health care staff who work there. The project was a qualitative case study of two genito-urinary clinics in central London. It was primarily ethnographic, involving two periods of non-participant observation, semi-structured interviews with staff and a small number of male clients ($n = 22$) in each clinic, together with analyses of documentary and historical data. It also included recruiting a small number of male readers of the popular and readily available *Men's Health* magazine, who were interviewed. It is a marker of the significance of the power of the hidden stories of male sexual desire and behaviour that a number of men from all over the UK were prepared to travel to London without payment, to be interviewed. In addition, the research involved historical analyses of the imagery of public health 'VD' (venereal diseases) campaigns and other visual representations of the nineteeth and twentieth centuries. The analyses of this thick, rich data provided the elements for a new sociology of sexual health and disease. However, what became increasingly apparent was the complexity of the medico-moral discourses, and the symbolic and cultural meanings surrounding sexuality, sexual diseases and their control. One useful way of understanding these processes is to explore the clinical encounter as a transaction, where the consumer of sex is then subject to a less welcome role as client of the expanding industry of sexual health.

The commodification of sexual health

Central to the dense web of medical/social/moral tensions in the clinical encounter is the emerging commodification of the clinic that reflects wider *consumer culture*. Smart (1993) summarized Bauman's argument that in consumer culture, consumption rather than work or productive activity has become the 'cognitive and moral focus of life, integrative bond of the society and the focus of systematic management'. Smart (1993: 64) goes on to suggest that:

> It is the pursuit of pleasure through the consumption of commodities that has become a necessity, rather than a self-denial or the deferring of gratification.

What is meant by this commodification of the clinic in the context of medical discourses? Smart's analysis can obviously relate to the apparent increasing consumption of the erotic by individuals. People may feel less inhibited by the moral constraints on sexual behaviour that historically were central to discourses of moral purity through self-denial. It might be that there were more taboos surrounding transgression of moral codes and that many, but by no means all, societies in the twenty-first century are more tolerant of sexual diversity, activities and sexual diseases.

If the consequences of this increased sexual consumption result in disease, then the clinic becomes simply a convenient 'one-stop' shop where technical treatments, dispensed apparently without moral judgement, may restore the individuals to continue their sexual activities. The clinic is thereby transformed from a dispensary to a series of products, constructed as a coherent centre for the distribution of treatments, education, health promotion and counselling while also retaining and extending its key role as a site of surveillance. It is tempting to view the clinic and health service generally like the wider economic, service sector as a prime example of McDonaldization (Ritzer 1983) where the rationalization of health care services is increasingly reconfigured within 'free market' principles. Ritzer argues how mass consumption is achieved through efficiency, calculability, predictability and control. The clinic is subject to these forces and is becoming an enterprise that has a series of sexual health products and services that are available to the individual. To this end, the clinic utilizes contemporary sexual imagery and values and is simply part of a complex set of elements in the commodification of sex. The STI clinic is now therefore continuous with, and contingent to, the individual's consumption of the erotic and its consequences.

It was also clear from the men in the study that attendance at the clinic was a complex interactional process where the client-as-consumer sought to acquire the best product (treatment, advice, counselling, reassurance) at least cost. The 'cost' to the consumer is the extent to which he must disclose personal, sexual information that does not cast him in a 'bad' light, such as using prostitutes or wilfully engaging in unsafe sex. Charles was an informed consumer, experienced in clinic attendance and confident in his role as an *out* gay man. However, when interviewed he was asked whether he always disclosed if he had unsafe sex, and he replied: 'No comment!'

> I don't mind talking about sexuality in the general sense and my sexual health going for blood tests, I suppose if I had known I had been 100 per cent safe there would have been no need for a blood test, so you can draw your own conclusions.

His reticence to disclose this 'new deviance' is common. As Ridge *et al.* (1997) argue, self-surveillance has been manipulated in gay culture to reinforce the belief that safer sex is 'the norm', despite the fact that the practice of unprotected anal intercourse is common.

The clinicians seek to professionalize the clinic by emphasizing both its medical and expert status. They attempt to 'neutralize' the stigma attached to 'VD', and extend the message of sexual health promotion through surveillance of the population. However, sexually transmitted infections often remain located in social discourses of guilt, contamination and impurity. There was evidence of different perceptions of stigma between different groups of men, for example straight and gay, that were highlighted by Alistair, a doctor in one clinic:

> In gay men there is a bit of dismissal of it [stigma] because it's a negative thing, because we're inverts or perverts or whatever already.

However, straight men and women definitely have a lot of guilt about coming here and infection relating to the genitals making them dirty, less desirable and so on. You've only got to look at their reaction to getting herpes on their genitals as opposed to a coldsore on the mouth. They are the same virus! It's a marker that they are a slut, that they are a dirty person.

The commodification of the clinic is also achieved through rationalizing services and efficiency inside the clinic by the use of appointment systems and the limiting of time that each client may be seen. The 'market' for their sexual health products might appear to be 'given' – that is, anyone with an infection will *naturally* seek treatment. The unhappy truth is that not every person who acquires an STI will seek treatment and might well continue in sexual activities with other people. However, the clinic diversifies through penetrating hitherto marginal groups seen as the vectors of disease such as prostitutes, drug users, young people, or through the emphasis on 'hidden' diseases with serious consequences such as chlamydia.

A further twist that is consistent with the commodification of health products within the capitalist model is the invention of 'new' pathologies as products. New taboos have developed, particularly around safer sex campaigns where in one clinic a brochure appeared inviting men to join a self-help counselling group if they feared that they were 'addicted' to unsafe sex. Of course, until a few years ago, and still for many people, unsafe sex is 'normal sex' that is now being pathologized.

Increasing markets and discreet consumers

The world-wide consumption of sexual health clinic services is huge and the global problem of STI is growing. In the UK there were particularly sharp rises in diagnoses of acute sexually transmitted infections between 1995 and 1999; diagnoses rose by 76 per cent for genital chlamydial infection, 55 per cent for gonorrhoea, 54 per cent for infectious syphilis and 20 per cent for genital warts (PHLS *et al.* 2000). The rises in acute sexually transmitted infections are likely to be associated with increasing unsafe sexual behaviour, particularly among young heterosexuals and men who have sex with men, although the substantial rise in genital chlamydial infection may also reflect increased testing for this infection. This highlights the scale of the problem of infection and provides the rationale for the expanding commodification of the STI clinic to meet demand and educate clients to minimize further risk.

Studies increasingly suggest that by the late 1990s there was less concern with maintaining safer sex practices among both young male heterosexual and gay populations (Durex Global Sex Survey 1997). However, around a quarter of a million men in the UK visited an STI clinic during the year

2000 but little appears to be known about these men, who are often characterized as shadowy figures. Negotiating access to the clinic for some men
requires discretionary strategies that echo Karp's (1973) phrase 'the management of public privacy' and the fear of 'seeing someone I know!'. Despite
attempts to destigmatize the clinics (Greenhouse 1996) and the increased
discussion of sexual issues in society, the attendees often carefully negotiate
a discreet entry to these stigmatizing clinics that are often located in the
least-loved parts of old hospitals.

Most men never experience such a clinical encounter while for others
attending the clinic is a routine part of the management of their sexual lives
and an essential element in the discourses of responsible sexual citizenship.
However, STI services do constitute a very significant degree of financial,
political and human involvement with sex and sexualities entering the clinical gaze. In the UK, there has been some research on the organization of
clinics (Allen and Hogg 1993) and a few studies explore consumer experiences (Evans and Farquhar 1996; Pryce 2000a) but little sociological
interest. In reality clinics may offer a range of services or 'clinics' that might
be offered in the evenings or for a couple of hours a week to particular
groups, such as sex industry workers. Surprisingly, however, little is known
of the pattern of use of clinics other than through statistical gathering of
population-based information by case. Nor has there been sociological
exploration of STI (as opposed to HIV/AIDS-related studies), other than
through surveys of what this STI encounter means to either the clients or
the professional health carers (Johnson et al. 1996).

Who are these clients and what do they do that is different from the men
who do not attend clinics? The National Survey (Johnson et al. 1994) did
suggest that in the UK the sexual behaviours of those who attended were
different from those who did not. Both male and female clients reported a
much higher level of heterosexual partners than non-attendees did. The attitudes reported by the National Survey suggest that, at a population level,
there is a low attendance by those with high-risk lifestyles (26.7 per cent men
who have sex with men; and 18.7 per cent who had paid for sex in the
previous year). Johnson et al. (1996: 202) argue that community studies
suggest that there are relatively low numbers of people with undiagnosed
syphilis or gonorrhoea in the population, with higher rates of herpes and
asymptomatic chlamydia. Thus, the clinics, they argue, provide an important
focus for health promotion programmes with high-risk attendees, but those
high-risk non-attendees require different strategies.

Consumerism, pragmatism and discretion management

Clinic attendance is not always driven by the need for treatment. It is a secret
site of confession, where even the information held on file by clinics cannot

be shared with a client's GP unless permission is given by the client (Robertson *et al.* 1989). A clinic is therefore a privileged place for resistance to other medico-legal discourses such as anonymity of treatment or HIV testing. From the consumer's perspective, it is safer and free from the inquiring gaze of insurance companies. For example, the role of the STI clinic was central in the 'to test or not to test' AIDS discourses in the mid and late 1980s (Davies *et al.* 1993: 95ff; Lupton *et al.* 1995). Clients may utilize the clinic strategically to clarify their HIV antibody status or reveal other potentially discrediting information with less fear of employers or the state and thereby circumvent their surveillance. Charles, a client at one clinic, goes on to describe:

> I basically started going to the pubs and clubs and wherever else gay men go to find sex. So from the point of view of going to a clinic I think what prompted that was I was going to make an application for insurance. I knew from being perfectly open about my sexuality in the past that insurance companies would send me off for an HIV test and God forbid if the HIV test was positive! Then I wanted to find out through a health adviser at a proper clinic with a sort of full pre- and post-counselling as opposed to having a very anonymous letter landing on my doorstep saying that my insurance application had been declined. Working in the financial services industry, I have only seen it once but I did not want that to happen to me. So, I wanted to find out through the more educated channels than a commercial organization. So I thought go for a blood test, the question of sexual health wasn't uppermost in my mind and I thought kill two birds with one stone and have a checkup at the same time.

While it is a public place, the clinic is concerned with the management of privacy, discretion, confidentiality, danger, anxiety, concealment, reassurance and disclosure. It is also a site of surveillence of particular populations such as gay men (Nardone *et al.* 1997) or the activities of prostitutes (Morse *et al.* 1992).

The Greek origin of the word 'clinic' is a 'public sanctuary for the voicing of trouble and the dispensing of relief' (Miller and Crabtree 1994: 349). This definition provides a useful metaphor that extends to the procedures that surround the organization and enactment of consultations, treatments and the eliciting of highly selective sexual histories as performative behaviours. The various notions of what is meant by 'public' permeate the acts of disclosure, both in the clinical performances by professionals and clients' stories of how the tensions around disclosure parallel the management of their own private/public sexualities. Through well-rehearsed dialogues, clients are required to recite their histories, behaviours and 'name the guilt', as one Health Adviser described it.

The public stage of the clinic is an arena in which powerful private discourses and tensions are evident. The ceremonial of biomedicine engages with the potentially subversive *erotic charge* brought to it by the clients. In the clinic, they are discrete and subject to ceremonials that ritually separates the individual actor from the bodily location to reduce the embarrassment and anxiety of clinical penetration of the urethra, rectum or vagina (Henslin 1971; Tunnadine 1980). As one nurse remarked when commenting on the power of the health professional's role in the clinic, 'we plant land-mines in their sex lives'. Interestingly, the deployment of such power must be swift. In terms of time the client spends with the doctor, Arya *et al.* (1994) suggested that in their study of a central urban clinic, this was the equivalent to an average of 20.3 minutes for a new patient and 13.9 minutes for an 'old' (i.e. previously registered) patient!

Clients attend clinics primarily because of symptoms of infection or the fear of infection resulting from an erotic encounter. A smaller number attend routinely as 'well-informed' patients aware of the potential risks of sexual activity. This group are regarded as 'good', 'well-motivated' and 'responsible' by clinic staff and it was generally assumed that this group comprised gay men, although some heterosexual men do attend routinely. An element in the discretionary process of clinic attendance is, of course, the choice of clinic. Hope and MacArthur (1997) surveyed users of five STI clinics in one city in the UK. Clients chose clinics based on recommendation (38.2 per cent) and proximity (36.4 per cent). Research in the clinic as a site that clients might choose for HIV testing, as opposed to anonymous HIV antibody testing services, suggests that each is likely to attract different groups (Hudson *et al.* 1997).

Among those who have a long history of STI and/or clinic attendance, a number of men reported that they had 'shopped around'. Guilio, like other men who are HIV positive, tends to attend one clinic for conditions related to the virus, and the STI clinic for any other sexual health issue. For most men, the decision whether to attend one or another clinic is clearly based on subjective responses consistent with modern notions of consumerist and lifestyle rhetoric. This includes making pragmatic choices that may in addition act as a form of resistance to the medical gaze. Gary, a young man who identified as bisexual, was clear in the criteria that he used when seeking clinic services.

INTERVIEWER: Did you make any choices about which clinic to attend in London?

GARY: Yes I did ... perhaps there should be a 'Good STI Clinic Guide'. ... I work on the principle that if I choose a clinic I must be able to park my car.

INTERVIEWER: So the choice of clinic is more determined by practical considerations like that rather than the reputation of the clinic?

GARY: Yes, I'm sure other people have other criteria. It's great that clinics specialize in gay people, younger people or bisexuals. It's great, and it is quite important to have a range of specialized services. I see that there is a clinic specializing in people under 26. If that had been around when I was 19 I would have definitely used it.

Gary's car as his 'own territory' is interesting in relation to clinic stories, while clearly outside the building it is both an important factor in selection of clinic and a symbolic means of retaining some control and ownership within a potentially disempowering situation. Graham, a married heterosexual man who had once had a 'holiday fling' with a woman from whom he had contracted an infection, suggested that while the impression of clinics was that they had formerly been for filthy and disgusting people he did not feel that himself. Furthermore, clinics were primarily concerned with enabling people to return to consuming sexual activities without moral or social judgement being made about them or their lifestyle:

GRAHAM: Did I feel filthy and disgusting? No, no I didn't. Really it's just like influenza. I never got into those ideas, I never got into the idea that she was filthy and disgusting because she had it. She was screwing around with a load of blokes, good on her, enjoy yourself while you can just be a bit more careful.

As a consumer of both sex and the clinic, Graham is demonstrating the overarching theme of contemporary sexual health. That, of course, reflects concerns that are more general where the individual is counselled to engage in more active personal risk assessment and management.

Similarly, another client had previously attempted to limit uncertainty by always having used private doctors for sexual health care because the problem was sex-related and he was concerned that seeing people he knew would compromise his social status, and therefore he sought anonymity. For David, a bisexual married man, the process of registering and acquiring a numerical identity had unforeseen consequences suggesting that registration at the clinic provided new, powerful impressions.

DAVID: I thought the first thing I must do when I get back is get tested. I looked around for a clinic and I wasn't sure how to go about it. I cannot remember now. How I did find out? Probably from the phone-book. I went on the Friday evening clinic ... I didn't know what to expect, although I thought it wouldn't be pleasant. I remember going into the clinic, they gave me a number – 3360. I didn't have to give my name.
INTERVIEWER: You remember the number!
DAVID: Yes 'cos I once tried to get cash out of my cash machine with it!

There is a tension between, on the one hand, the urgent desire for comfort and relief from the stress of 'contamination' and, on the other, ensuring confidentiality. Other men also employed purposeful strategies to ensure anonymity for insurance testing purposes and to set personal agendas. The criteria for selecting one clinic or another are sometimes complex. Charles is a gay man but not 'out' to his family or work colleagues:

CHARLES: I suppose ... I went to that clinic because it is very close to an HIV/AIDS clinic and clearly there was a lot of overlap between staff, and because a large proportion of the visitors are gay it is very gay friendly compared to St Simon's. The receptionist clearly has two windows on either side of her area, one for the women and one for the men ... and a greater balance of the men at St Simon's I would say are straight than my experience tells me was the case at the other clinic.

Men who were developing their sexual careers and managing their sexual identities often mentioned this concern with gender and orientation of staff. These included men who usually identified as heterosexual but who routinely sought to have sex with men while commuting between work and home, or men who expressed an erotic aesthetic through body piercing or tattoos that most of the time remained hidden so they could retain 'respectable' jobs.

Consumption and its discontents

The male ambivalence surrounding sexuality, health and the body of course results in many men being very reluctant consumers. There are some diseases and conditions which, although not sexually acquired, can affect men's sexualities, but are not the primary reason for men seeking medical opinion or treatment at an STI clinic rather than from a GP. These conditions potentially create stigmatizing threats to men, their bodies and require discretionary strategies in seeking medical consultation. For example, Gordon (1995: 246ff) has explored testicular cancer and the danger this poses to hegemonic notions of men's sex role, thereby highlighting the construction of masculine identity and suggesting why so many men are reluctant to seek medical help.

Historically, a number of factors have been proposed to explain why many men find attending the clinic, or indeed any medical examination, a problematic experience. Reid and Fine (1992: 132ff) usefully identify four factors which may inhibit intimacy among males: competition; homophobia; aversion to vulnerability and openness; and lack of role models. In popular magazines such as *Men's Health*, male anxieties seem to be focused on sexual performance and represented within the context of competitiveness in lifestyle and success. Such representations also reflect latent homophobia, such as one article in *Men's Health* (October 1999) that addressed the protocol of using public toilets so that unintended sexual signals could be avoided. More sociological evidence is provided by Holland *et al.* (1996: 147) whose research revealed an emphasis on 'performance' in male narratives that was largely absent in similar interviews with young women.

While the central concern in male sexual anxiety is commonly assumed to be intercourse performance, other anxieties include the public exposure of the genitals and rectum, penis size and genital abnormalities. However, men in the study suggested that exposing the genitals might create less anxiety in the STI clinic compared with GP consultations. Nevertheless, the performance centred locus of male sexual belief is profound. Anxieties focused on performance permeate modes of male social interaction as well as the individual imagination, from the bedroom to the clinical examination.

To some extent, this might be justifiable, for example, in that erectile dysfunction may affect 10 per cent of men (Liando *et al.* 1996: 24). The loss of performance eroding self-image, reproductive function or the notion of being a 'real man' is at the heart of late modern discourses about men, male identities and masculinities. Admitting impotence, and having to display the penis as the source of betrayal in a clinical examination, profoundly destabilizes hegemonic masculinity. The paradox is that the clinic treats the unwanted consequences of sexual encounters while, for some men who desperately seek penetrative erotic activity, the same clinic is the site of their confession of 'failure'. A central problem then for clinics is how to market their services to consumers who would really prefer not to have to utilize them! Apart from the relatively small number of regular clients at each clinic, clinic attendance for most men is unwelcome, infrequent and largely driven by need.

The experience for many men is that their sexual and reproductive body is less medically observed compared with women who are the object of overt surveillance from childhood onwards. However, there are now also increased representations and consumption of the exposed, unclothed, eroticized male body in advertising, the media and the construction of the 'new' man (Nixon 1996). In the constructions of the hegemonic male body and identity, there has also been a relative lack of vocabulary in male culture to describe sexual function and its emotional or psychosocial context. This relationship between the emotions and the body is at the centre of contemporary discourses (Petersen 1998), and may explain the rupture between men's sexual practices and their ability simply to describe them. The sexual stories and language used by men particularly with other men is often coded because of constraints on male intimacy and to do otherwise subverts established rules of dominant masculine culture. Evidence from both the literature (Komarovsky 1974; Aukett *et al.* 1988; Reid and Fine 1992) and the men in the research, suggests that men are more likely to disclose intimate and personal information to women than to another male. For gay men interviewed in the study, the majority stated that they would prefer to see a gay male doctor or a woman doctor with heterosexual male doctors as the least favourite option. However, for heterosexual male clients it seemed that the gender of the staff was less important than professional competence and speedy service!

The lay histories and fables of the 'pox', 'clap' and other sexually transmitted diseases permeate men's expectation of clinic attendance with the painful treatments (punishment) and potentially stigmatizing consequences of going to the clinic. In no other place, except within sex acts, is the male body, especially the sexualized male body, under such scrutiny. In the clinic, it is exposed, viewed, touched and penetrated within an arena (apparently) devoid of the erotic but filled with the incitement to talk about sex and charged with the potential danger of sexual expression. This clearly (re)creates ambivalence in those paid to provide health care for men. However, the literature suggests that the clinical gaze extends beyond the clinic itself to locate, chart and collect information about the sexual networks and relationships within populations and communities. This process, as Armstrong (1983; 1993; 1995) has described, positions the client's sexual experiences, identity and life outside the clinic as both continuous with, and reconstructed by, the gaze inside the clinic. How then is the individual client recruited and deployed in this project of sexual health commodification?

The deployment of the active patient as consumer

The clinical examination is one key element in the process of recruiting the active patient. I have suggested elsewhere (Pryce 2000b) that in the process of seeking treatment, the client's stories are clearly not 'objective'. They conform to the ceremonial of clinical consultation and examination. Social regulation is at the heart of the clinical dialogue, whereby both staff and client negotiate the script of complex interactions in clinical encounters (Heath 1984). It is clear that the interrogation by the professional of the patient/client's sexual behaviours contravenes everyday conversational conventions because of the extent of disclosure about personal behaviour and practices. Thus, in sexual matters it extends the medical consultation beyond the comfortable clinical territory for doctors, nurses and clients.

In tracing the later emergence of the surveillance in public health and health promotion Armstrong (1983: 12) argued that,

the outcry against VD in the early part of the 20th C. was not only a manifestation of moral outrage but also of latent surveillance possibilities: the path of venereal diseases throughout the community traced the threads which linked one person intimately with another. The dangers of venereal disease could be used as a means of observing behaviour, educating thoughts and teaching contacts.

The deployment of sexual health regimes operates through the individual as 'the active patient' (Armstrong 1993: 61); that is, central to the construction of the client as consumer. This active patient role extends to the consumption and practices of sex and sexual identities. It is woven into the construction of cultural associations between sex and shame, impurity, danger and risk (Ridge *et al.* 1997). The clinic is not the only site where the discursive formations of sexualities and medicine interpenetrate and the government of sexual health is deployed. Consumption of popular culture, the media as well as legal and political factors also reinforce individualistic responsibility for sexuality and health. When discussing 'safe sex culture' within the gay scene in Australia, Ridge *et al.* (1997: 149) argue that although assumed a 'norm', for men practising condom-unprotected anal intercourse, self-monitoring has engendered guilt and shame. The social histories and mythologies of sex and sexual diseases permeate many social and sexual activities.

The stories of sexual careers are interwoven with such discourses and issues of purity and danger, not least when considered in relation to clinic professionals. Staff must balance their own roles and desires as sexual citizens and sexual health professionals. What is 'cool' and liberal in the clinic may change when they themselves must become client/consumers! One nurse revealed the difficulty of disclosing this at work:

INTERVIEWER: What stops you standing up and saying (you have herpes too)?
JOSIE: The fact that I caught it people just go (gasps) like 'God, you know, she's got herpes, she's a nurse, she should know better!'. I'm just worried about what people think about me, basically being judgemental about me.
INTERVIEWER: Even in a clinic that specialized in sexually transmitted diseases?
JOSIE: Yeah, even here!

The commodification of the clinic is further developed through the array of health promotion literature, counselling, outreach and specialist activities that target particular client markets. These include male and female prostitutes, young gay men or rape victims. The professionals may have experiential and ideological 'streetwise' awareness of categories and practices of sexual groups. Some men who regularly attend are adept at the consumerist game whereby honour is served 'by rendering unto Caesar ...'. In other words, the client plays the game of docile but knowledgeable consumer of services while simultaneously pursuing and refining his 'unsafe' erotic desires and practices.

Conclusion

I have proposed that historically the acquisition and treatment of sexually transmitted infections has been socially problematic. However, it is remarkable to consider how quickly the stigmatizing experience of the 'VD' clinic is being transfigured into a service that is consistent with other forms of health practices. In addition, there is a growing population who may require clinical services. As consumers, the population is expected to be increasingly educated about the precautions required to avoid disease and pregnancy, and the dangers of unsafe sexual activities in a culture that is increasingly immersed in calculations of risk. Similarly, changing social mores and attitudes have meant that in many societies it is now acceptable to talk more openly about sex and sexual infections, to 'tolerate' sexual differences and to challenge heteronormative assumptions of sexual identity and gender roles.

It is not surprising that the clinic has been transformed to fulfil the role of providing relatively stigma-free sexual health services within a social climate of increasing consumerism. The reconstruction of the clinic into a series of commodities – treatment and diagnosis, education, public health and surveillance – is thereby entirely consistent with the need to engage with the increasing commodification of sex itself. This response to the consumerization of society, with its greater expectations of services and with individuals who have learnt to be more assertive in the demand for 'choice', client centred, 'holistic' and convenient services is being addressed in many aspects of health care. The STI clinic provides a prime example of how this commodification takes place and how it both reflects and shapes public opinion as an expectation. An example of the changing professional norms is the privileging of confessional talk about sexual behaviour and identity, and the 'up front' use of lay sexual terminology and 'street-cred' knowledge of sexual practices and spaces. It is also apparent in the identification and provision of 'niche' markets for specific groups such as survivors of rape or young gay and lesbian clients.

Clinical commodification may not be welcomed by some health professionals who might see it as an erosion of professional status and resent the increasing consumerist strategic use of power. In addition, some clients may remain uncomfortable about disclosing 'private' information, or might be reluctant to abstain from sex during a course of treatment or may not attend at all despite the abundant evidence of infection. Indeed, many clients are able to use services while not fully 'confessing' and selectively use services, such as men who continue to have unprotected sex – they wish treatment for infection but the rationalities they employ when engaging in sex are not those of 'safer sex'.

In this chapter I have tried to suggest that the overarching processes of commodification result from a cluster of economic, social and moral 'drivers' within societies that are reconfiguring and extending contemporary ideas of 'what is health?'. In this regard, individual citizens are being recruited into the project of monitoring their own health and are increasingly held responsible for maintaining healthy lifestyle regimes as 'active patients'. As the 'active patient', the individual becomes consumer both of sex itself and the services that educate and provide treatment if infection results from the encounter. Clearly, the business of the clinic must be to accept the role of provider and use the language and the media of consumption to ensure that their product, the sexual health commodities, reach the biggest audience most effectively. The emergence of the contemporary sexual health clinic as a provider of services that are continuous with sexual consumption, and the beliefs, behaviours and practices of the individual client, may therefore be a marker of its success!

References

Allen, I. and Hogg, D. (1993) *Work Roles and Responsibilities in Genitourinary Medicine Clinics*, London: Policy Studies Institute.

Armstrong, D. (1983) *Political Anatomy of the Body: Medical Knowledge in Britain in the Twentieth Century*, Cambridge: Cambridge University Press.

—— (1993) 'From clinical gaze to regime of total health', in A. Beattie, M. Gott, L. Jones and M. Sidell (eds) *Health and Well Being: A Reader*, Basingstoke: Macmillan and Open University Press.

—— (1995) 'The rise of surveillance medicine', *Sociology of Health and Illness*, 17, 3: 393–404.

Arya, O.P., Davies, J., Fagan, M., Sullivan, B. and Evans, C. (1994) 'Doctor time requirement for patient consultation in genitourinary medicine clinics', *Genitourinary Medicine*, 70: 339–40.

Aukett, R., Ritchie, J. and Mill, K. (1988) 'Gender differences in friendship patterns', *Sex Roles*, 19: 57–66.

Davies, P., Hickson, F.C.I. Weatherburn, P. and Hunt, A.J. (1993) *Sex, Gay Men and AIDS*, London: The Falmer Press.

Durex (1997) *Durex Global Sex Survey 1997*, London: London International Group.

Evans, D. and Farquhar, C. (1996) 'An interview based approach to seeking user views in genitourinary medicine', *Genitourinary Medicine*, 72: 223–6.

Foucault, M. (1991) 'Governmentality', in G. Burchill, C. Gordon and P. Miller (eds) *The Foucault Effect: Studies in Governmentality*, Hemel Hempstead: Harvester Wheatsheaf, pp. 87–104.

Gordon, D.F. (1995) 'Testicular cancer and masculinity', in D. Sabo and D.F. Gordon (eds) *Men's Health and Illness: Gender, Power and the Body*, Thousand Oaks, CA: Sage.

Greenhouse, P. (1996) 'Destigmatising sexual health clinics', *British Journal of Sexual Medicine*, 23, 5: 13–16.

Heath, C. (1984) 'Participation in the medical consultation: the co-ordination of verbal and non-verbal behaviour between the doctor and patient', *Sociology of Health and Illness*, 6, 3: 311–38.

Henslin, J.M. (ed.) (1971) 'Dramaturgical desexualization: the sociology of the vaginal examination', in *Studies in the Sociology of Sex*, New York: Appleton-Century-Crofts.

Holland, J., Ramazangoglu, C. and Thomson, R. (1996) 'In the same boat? The gendered (in)experience of first heterosex', in D. Richardson (ed.) *Theorising Heterosexuality: Telling it Straight*, Buckingham: Open University Press.

Hope, V.D. and MacArthur, C. (1997) 'Acceptability of clinics for sexually transmitted diseases among users of the "gay scene" in the West Midlands', *Genitourinary Medicine*, 73: 299–302.

Hudson, M.M.T., Nelson, W.L., Ronalds, C.J., Anderson, J. and Jeffries, D.J. (1997) 'HIV antibody testing: genito-urinary clinic or additional site same-day testing service', *AIDS Care*, 9, 2: 209–15.

Johnson, A.M., Wadsworth, J., Wellings, K. and Field, J. (1994) *Sexual Attitudes and Lifestyle*, Oxford: Blackwell.

—— (1996) 'Who goes to sexually transmitted disease clinics? Results from a national population survey', *Genitourinary Medicine*, 72, 3: 197–202.

Karp, D.A. (1973) 'Hiding in pornographic bookstores: a reconsideration of the nature of urban anonymity', in *Urban Anthropology*, 1, 4: 427–52.

Komarovsky, M. (1974) 'Patterns of self-disclosure of male undergraduates', *Journal of Marriage and the Family*, 36: 677–86.

Liando, M., Glover, L. and Abel, P. (1996) 'Erectile difficulties', *British Journal of Sexual Medicine*, 23, 3: 24–5.

Lupton, D. (1995) *The Imperative of Health: Public Health and the Regulated Body*, London: Sage.

Lupton, D., McCarthy, S. and Chapman, S. (1995) 'Panic bodies: discourses on risk and HIV antibody testing', *Sociology of Health and Illness*, 17, 1: 89–108.

McClean, H.L., Reid, M. and Scoular, A. (1995) ' "Healthy alliances?": other sexual health services and their views of genitourinary medicine', *Genitourinary Medicine*, 71, 6: 396–9.

McKeganey, N. and Barnard, M. (1996) *Sex Work on the Streets*, Buckingham: Open University Press.

Miller, W.L. and Crabtree, B.F. (1994) 'Clinical research', in N. Denzin and Y.S. Lincoln (eds) *Handbook of Qualitative Research*, Thousand Oaks: Sage.

Morse, E.V., Simon, P.M., Balson, M. and Osofsky, J. (1992) 'Sexual behavior patterns of customers of male street prostitutes', *Archives of Sexual Behaviour*, 21, 4: 347–57.

Nardone, A., Mercey, D.E. and Johnson, A.M. (1997) 'Surveillance of sexual behaviour among homosexual men in a central London health authority', *Genitourinary Medicine*, 73: 198–202.

Nettleton, S. (1992) *Power, Pain and Dentistry*, Buckingham: Open University Press.

—— (1995) *The Sociology of Health and Illness*, Cambridge: Polity Press.

Nixon, S. (1996) *Hard Looks*, London: UCL Press.

Petersen, A. (1998) *Unmasking the Masculine: 'Men' and 'Identity' in a Sceptical Age*, London: Sage.

Petrak, J.A., Skinner, C.J. and Claydon, E.J. (1995) 'The prevalence of sexual assault in a genitourinary medicine clinic: service implications', *Genitourinary Medicine*, 71: 98–102.

PHLS, DHSS and PS, Scottish ISD(D)5 Collaborative Group (2000) *Trends in Sexually Transmitted Infections in the United Kingdom, 1990–1999*, London: Public Health Laboratory Service.

Pryce, A. (2000a) *Eros Beyond the Clinical Gaze: Elements for a Sociology of Sexually Transmitted Disease*, Portsmouth: Nursing Praxis International.

—— (2000b) 'Does your mother know you are heterosexual?': discretion management and resistance of the erotic in the genitourinary clinic', *Critical Public Health*, 10, 3: 1–17.

Reid, H.M. and Fine, G.A. (1992) 'Self-disclosure in men's friendships: variations associated with intimate relations', in P.M. Nardi (ed.) *Men's Friendships*, Newbury Park: Sage.

Ridge, D., Minichiello, V. and Plummer, D. (1997) 'Queer connections: community, "the Scene" and an epidemic', *Journal of Contemporary Ethnography*, 26, 2: 146–81.

Ritzer, G. (1983) *The McDonaldization of Society: An Investigation into the Changing Character of Contemporary Social Life*, Thousand Oaks: Pine Forge Press.

Robertson, D.H.H., McMillan, A. and Young, H. (1989) *Clinical Practice in Sexually Transmissible Diseases* (2nd edn), Edinburgh: Churchill Livingstone.

Smart, B. (1993) *Postmodernity*, London: Routledge.

Tunnadine, P. (1980) 'The role of genital examination in psychosexual medicine', *Clinics in Obstetrics and Gynaecology*, 7, 2: 283–91.

Turner, B.S. (1984) *The Body and Society*, Oxford: Blackwell.

Chapter 10

Young people, drug use and the consumption of health

Elizabeth Ettorre and Steven Miles

Introduction

Both sociological and popular conceptions of 'youth' tend to portray young people either as 'victims' of social and economic restructuring or as troublesome rebels liable to succumb to the excesses of drug and alcohol dependency and violence (Miles 2000). Both of these positions constitute gross oversimplifications. Young people are active, creative negotiators of the relationship between structure and agency (see McDonald 1999). This creativity is expressed most clearly in the context of consumption: the socio-cultural arena within which the young are, or at least should be, able to navigate through the uncertainties of social change. The problem with discourses on youth consumption, however, is that these tend to focus on young people as risk-takers (Plant and Plant 1992) or as risky consumers which thereby reinforces a pathological model of youth (Miles 2000). Discussions of young people's health suffer from the same problem (Brannen *et al.* 1994).

Our chapter illustrates the limitations of this approach to health consumption *vis-à-vis* drug services which are striking for their failure to account for strategic if not pleasurable aspects of young people's patterns of consumption. We are primarily concerned with young people's consumption of health, drugs and drug services in Britain. We divide our discussion into two main sections. In the first, we focus on the problems inherent in portraying young people both as 'victims' and as 'consumers'. In section two, we look at a case study of young people as consumers of drugs and drug services. Our main contention, drawn from the work of Griffin (1997), is that young people's lives are all about occupying distinct social spaces in the routes of production, reproduction and consumption, all of which are located in specific gender, sex, class and race contexts. We contend further that in order to have a clear picture of young people's consumption of drugs and drug services, we must understand their lives from this viewpoint. In short, priority needs to be given to the development of a 'youth-sensitive' approach to the young as consumers of these drug services.

Young people as 'victims' and as consumers

Young people as 'victims'

The sociology of youth is dominated by an orthodoxy in which the agency of young people is largely neglected. Discussions of young people's transitions are concerned with aspects of unemployment, education and training (e.g. Roberts 1995). In doing so, these tend to focus on broad economic trends which determine how easy it is for the young to reach adulthood. This reflects the argument that traditional routes into adulthood have, in recent years, been problematized. Discussions of the 'transition' focus on the ways in which social structures affect the development of the young. Within this discourse there is very little room for discussion of the ways in which young people actively negotiate with dominant power structures. Consumption represents one means of doing so.

In this context, Rutherford (1997) discusses the emergence in 1990s Britain of an increasingly disadvantaged youth and, in particular, homeless youth, who symbolize the way in which the decline in welfare and changes in the job market appear to have affected the young more than any other social group. Young people are usually the most vulnerable social group to be affected by social and economic change. This approach to what it means to be a young person is very much a by-product of the 1980s. For instance, Cashmore (1984) describes a world in which the young have 'no future' and in which they are resigned to having few ambitions, limited horizons and almost no prospects. Young people are in a crisis inasmuch as rising unemployment, welfare and education cuts, and a decade of right-wing government are apparently taking their toll (Griffin 1997). From this point of view young people are wounded by, if not victims of, social change.

Alongside this vision of victimhood, many authors have also pointed out that the young are a barometer of social change. In addition, Jones and Wallace (1992) note that the young might equally be conceptualized as an index of social *ills*. This latter proposition may well be the case. However, to accept this unconditionally simply serves to underestimate the complexity of young people's experience. Young people are more than passive casualties of unemployment trends, drug misuse and problems associated with teenage pregnancy. Young people are not simply all about the melodrama of sub-cultural life or the terrors of youth crime, drug addiction and alcohol consumption. In many ways the young are an index of social *norms*, and their patterns of consumption constitute the playing out of such norms.

For too long sociology has neglected what we describe as 'mainstream youth', in favour of a sociology of the melodramatic. This focus on the 'problematic' aspects of youth has discouraged reflexive approaches to young people's actual experiences of social change. Jones (1995) discusses the emergence of 'the youth problem', and, in doing so, she points out that the focus appears to be on the problems young people seem to pose for society, as opposed to the problems society creates for the young. She therefore considers the suggestion that, 'In a world in which increased individual choice and consumer rights are stressed, the choices and rights of young people are ignored' (Jones 1995: 5). Young people are simply not seen to be positive contributors to society in general. Indeed, from this point of view, as Jones notes, any contributions they do make would tend to be in the private world of family life, and, as a result, the young are not seen to be the responsibility of the state. On the one hand, the problems of the young tend to be seen as self-inflicted; on the other, because they are not yet adults, some may view them as not wholly responsible for their 'deviant behaviour'. Nevertheless, 'youth' problems tend to be seen as personal failures, while this sense of personal failure is magnified by the uncertainties of social change. The argument we want to put forward is that young people's patterns of consumption – in this instance, drugs – represents a cultural manifestation of their experience of such uncertainty. In other words, young people's consumption of drugs represents an active expression of their relationship with social structure, and, indeed, risk (Miles 2000). The way in which drug services deal with aspects of young people's drug consumption should, therefore, reflect situations in which the young are more than simply victims of social change. Awareness of risk as a common part of adolescent life (Collison 1996), and of young people as consumers of risk, should be generated within services that are supposed to be empowering in nature.

Young people, risk and consumption

This vision of young people as 'victims' is mirrored by an equally negative media-driven notion of 'youth'. As Griffin (1997) notes, there has been a series of moral panics over youth by adults in academia, government and social and welfare work. These panics have centred on issues such as teenage pregnancy, food and youth crime and, of course, drug use. Young people are therefore characterized as 'risky consumers'.

In all of these panics, specific groups of young are singled out for attention, and the focus of concern often deals with some aspect of young people's relationship to the cycle of production, reproduction and consumption. 'Problem teens' appear as a source of (adult) concern over (specific) young people's disordered relationship with consumption (e.g. drug use and food), reproduction (e.g. 'teen mothers') and/or production, which usually refers to the transition from education to the job market – e.g. slackers, youth crime (Griffin 1997: 8).

The relationship between young people's experience of social structure and consumption is therefore symbiotic. In a sense, this relationship is an expression of young people's positioning within the risk society. Many authors have pointed out that social change is such that the individual has been removed from traditional commitments and support relationships to the extent that:

> The place of traditional ties and social forms (i.e. social class, nuclear family) is taken by secondary agencies and institutions, which stamp the biography of the individual and make that person dependent upon fashions, social policy, economic cycles and markets, contrary to the image of individual control which establishes itself in consciousness.
>
> (Beck 1992: 131)

Many authors therefore see the young as especially vulnerable to the heightened sense of risk and the individualization of experience that has characterized the move towards 'high modernity'. In short, journeys into adulthood are becoming increasingly precarious. Whereas in the past young people would have navigated a way through to adulthood with the help of traditional support mechanisms such as the family, community and religion, nowadays any tough choices or decisions about the future fall squarely on young people's own individualized shoulders (Furlong and Cartmel 1997). Thus, consumption represents an arena where the young construct lifestyles within which they can live and negotiate with aspects of the risk society.

The key question arising from any discussion of young people, as consumers, is the extent to which consumerism provides the young with the sorts of freedoms to which they might aspire. Again, there is a tendency to see the young as a highly vulnerable sector of the population, easily persuaded, for example, by the superficialities of advertising (see Nava and Nava 1990). A world has apparently been created in which young people are programmed to consume. In short, consumption is a distraction that blinds young people from the dominant power structures that ensure their impotence. Indeed, the rebelliousness of young people is, from this point of view, a thing of the past; the young are far more likely to positively embrace the values of a consumer culture. Young people are struggling to assert their own sense of identity on the area of their lives over which they appear to have most control. Young people may express their identities through consumption, but ultimately such identities can never be expressed entirely freely. Consumption undoubtedly provides a key arena in which the young can begin to explore themselves. In a sense, then, youth is defined *through* consumption and, as such, it certainly should not be assumed that young people's consumption habits are uncritical in nature. The pleasures the young experience through drug consumption represent more than just an 'escape' but an active comment on the tensions and uncertainties that characterize the experience of youth at the beginning of the twenty-first century (see Miles *et al.* 1997).

Young people as consumers of health

Before going on to look more specifically at the question of young people as consumers of drugs and drug services, it is important to consider more closely young people as consumers of health. Again, there is an over-whelming emphasis in the literature on young people's propensity to take risks with their health. Montgomery and Schoon (1997) point out that social disadvantage is associated with a proclivity to take health risks. Furthermore, Ensign and Gittelsohn (1998) note that while disadvantaged homeless young people are aware of their health needs, these are shaped, on a daily basis by risky social contexts. In seeking to address the nature of young people's health in their mid-20s, Montgomery and Schoon (1997) go on to discuss three kinds of health-related behaviour, namely weight, drinking and smoking. This sort of an approach is typical of discussions into young people's health, insofar as the focus here is actually on the *poor* state of young people's health. Young people are again pathologized because they are *assumed* to be unhealthy by implication, precisely because their lifestyles apparently predispose them to poor health.

A focus on young people's risky lifestyles creates the impression that the young are socially problematic. For instance, Furlong and Cartmel (1997) argue that the uncertainties of social change have left the young in a situa-tion in which a sense of having no future has led to an increased incidence of mental illness, eating disorders, suicide and attempted suicide. In short, youth is an increasingly stressful experience and young people are increas-ingly vulnerable as a result. Thus, Smith and Rutter (1995) argue that psychosocial disorders have become much more prevalent among young people since the mid-1980s. As such, Burke et al. (1990) describe adolescence as a 'window of risk' (see Furlong and Cartmel 1997: 67). Furlong and Cartmel go on to argue that the age distribution of eating disorders reflects the impact of key transitions. The incidence of eating disorders peaks at the ages of 14 and 18, coinciding with the ages of sexual maturation and transi-tion into adulthood through employment and education.

The problem with any discussion of young people's health, however, is that very little attention is paid to young people as consumers of health *provision*. That young people are seen to be risk-takers undermines any claim they might have to adequate and sensible 'youth' centred provision. Young people are viewed as irresponsible and therefore potentially unde-serving consumers. The onus in Furlong and Cartmel's discussion, for instance, is on young people as risk-takers: as smokers, drinkers, drug users and sexual experimenters. Young people's experience of health is therefore portrayed, in a sense, as deviant. The priority here is on the potentially unhealthy behaviours in which the young are involved, rather than any posi-tive, healthy aspects of young people's lifestyles, such as the consumption of organic foods. Yes, young people are vulnerable and such vulnerability is a reflection of social change, but the end result of this focus on young people's health behaviours is that the young are passive recipients of such changes and not active or creative consumers. They take health risks and those health risks are largely socially unacceptable.

Our concern here is that a fundamental change needs to occur in the way in which young people's health is perceived. Young people continue to be pathologized in the sense that any discussion of young people's health focuses on young people's lifestyles. From this point of view the implication is that the young are the 'victims' of their own irresponsibility. In contrast, we prefer to conceptualize young people as active agents who use modes of consumption as a means of making sense of a rapidly changing world and, at times, as ways of seeking pleasure.

Young people as consumers of drugs and drug services

In the remainder of this article we want to suggest that if the young are victims at all, at least within the context of health, they are victims of the irresponsibility of health and social welfare *producers*. Young people's lifestyles are at least partially a product of the way in which they have been pathologized as a group. Only by focusing on young people as deserving citizens and thus, worthy consumers of health services can positive steps be taken to improve both the nature of health provision and young people's consumption of it. In other words, rather than prioritizing melodramatic aspects of young people's unhealthy behaviour through risky consumption, there needs to be more of an emphasis on the ways in which young people's health needs are being met.

Following on from discussions presented in the first section of our chapter, we focus on a case study of the young as consumers of drugs and drug services. We illustrate that the actual providers of health provision are themselves operating according to a pathological model of youth, to the extent that any freedoms we might associate with young people's consumption of health provision are largely superficial in nature. In effect, the rhetoric we associate with the freedom of the consumer has only served to wed the young to notions of victimhood which, in turn, actively legitimize pathological notions of youth.

We will look specifically at how young people's drug use is viewed as 'unhealthy' behaviour – a type of risky consumption and an emblem of unsuccessful socialization. Our focus then shifts and we look at young people's consumption of drug services. Here, our assumption is that drug services are founded on a pathological model of youth, which limits the scope and freedom associated with young people's consumption of healthy lifestyles and serves to control and restrain youth as disruptive consumers and 'dispossessed' citizens.

Young people's drug use as 'unhealthy' behaviour

As noted above, the pathological model of youth is grounded ontologically in the 'youth as a distinct stage in the lifecourse' viewpoint. For example, if old age can be represented as 'bodies in decline' (Featherstone and Hepworth 1998), youth can be represented as 'bodies in ascent'. The view that youthful bodies occupy distinct social spaces in the circuit of production, reproduction and consumption, all located in specific gender, sex, class and race contexts (Griffin 1997), is absent in the pathological model of youth. Why is young people's consumption of illegal drugs viewed as particularly unhealthy? One answer could be that consumption of drugs hinders the youthful 'body in ascent'. Of course, when healthy, youthful bodies are represented on the social landscape of 'normality', these bodies are most certainly 'ascending' as drug free. But, the main argument used for the prevention of young people's drug use tends to be centred on the reduction of harm – a notion that is equally applied to adults.

The reduction of harm to the individual user/consumer has been the basis of the British approach to drug control for much of the twentieth century (Berridge 1998). However, the reduction of harm to the young has particular social implications, given that drug use has become endemic and viewed as an inevitable part of youth culture by contemporary researchers (Blackman 1996; Parker et al. 1998). Indeed, the work of the Schools Education Unit (Balding 2000) exposes the fact that drugs are embedded in our youth cultures, as many adolescents have knowledge of illegal drug cultures, if not first-hand experience of drug use. Thus, the picture is one of most, if not all, young people being 'at risk' of consuming drugs and those young people that do consume drugs as being, in effect, 'duped' by the drug culture.

This picture fits well within the pathological model of youth because within this model young people's trouble-making or unhealthy behaviour is viewed as expected or inevitable. However, young people's trouble-making or 'unhealthy' behaviour will only be tolerated when these are limited by the discourses of care and control, imposed upon them by their elders (i.e. parents, society, etc.) or at least by those seen as outside of themselves. As the young attempt to manage their transitions to adulthood, they are in turn managed by those limiting discourse of care and control, operating as 'youth targeting' treatment regimes. Nevertheless, as consumers of both legal and illegal drugs, young people do not see drug use as a 'single issue' (Teeman et al. 1999), neither do they necessarily link drugs with unhealthy behaviour, as their parents, teachers or policy-makers do. Rather, for them, drug use is a piece of 'hedonistic/functional consumption' (Brain, Parker and Carnwath 2000); it can be *fun* (Henderson 1999). Thus, young people's psychoactive repertoires (i.e. use of alcohol, tobacco or illegal drugs) become framed within the context of consumption decisions – not necessarily decisions about their health (Brain et al. 2000).

In this atmosphere, moral panics are bound to gain ascendancy. This is not because young people ignore health or healthy lifestyles in their drug consumption decisions; rather, the adult world of the media, policy-makers and treaters view young people's drug consumption as being embodied in their pleasure-seeking or hedonistic lifestyles. This rather superficial view paints a picture of disaffected youth distancing themselves from the safeguards of public health. Young people who use drugs are seen to privilege consumption and pleasure over abuse. In this way, they appear to take 'health versus harm' out of the drugs equation. A danger arises that their ritualized cultures could become the targets of moral crusaders, seeking to justify policies of neglect, segregation, containment, separation and confinement (MacGregor 1999). If this occurs, the young could become 'victims' of these harsh, unsympathetic policies.

Young people's drug use as risky behaviour/consumption

Emerging from the drug policy in the USA, concepts such as 'dangerous classes' and 'War on Drugs' and a philosophy of 'zero tolerance' are sold regularly on the global drug policy market. One only has to attend international drug policy conferences to hear these sorts of mantras coming from US drug experts. These policy pundits who successfully sell this discourse of drugs on the global policy market help to construct specific configurations and treatment regimes about illegal drugs which actively impact upon the lives of drug users everywhere. While the overwhelming, global, public discourse on drugs is that it is a commodity that needs control, if not obliteration, the picture is one of risky products being consumed in cultural markets in which the calculus of risk varies by age, class, gender, race and even nationality.

Already viewed 'at risk' by society at some level, young people receive the message that drug use is a dangerous commodity. But, they may consider it to be a risk worth taking, given that, for some groups of 'troubled teens', they are in any case viewed as having a disordered relationship with consumption (Griffin 1997). While their involvement in drug use can be seen in the light of disordered patterns of consumption, young people who are drug users become disordered consumers. Their drug use becomes characterized as a potentially risky behaviour (e.g. drug use) linked with a specific form of risky consumption – 'consumption of risk products, drugs that act as social distinguishers' (Bunton and Burrows 1995: 218). These young people are viewed as risky, disordered consumers in an illegal drug market constructed as endemic in the urban economy as well as in the context of youth culture (Blackman 1997).

Here, the argument is not whether or not these young people take drugs. Rather, the point is that as consuming, embodied subjects, young people are 'socialized into society', while, at the same time, their drug consumption styles become normalized within the arena of disordered consumption

(Parker *et al.* 1998). While the risk calculus between hedonism and health draws a fine line (Measham *et al.* 2000), young people create cultures of survival (Blackman 1997). Disordered consumption in the form of both recreational and non-recreational drug use may be embedded in youth cultures. However, young people's consumption is not only what South and Teeman (1999) refer to as a 'smorgasbord of drugs' but also survival strategies that are constructed, managed and acted out in these enduring cultures. If drug use is *the* form of risky consumption for young people, it is logical that the experience of this type of consumption is as much about social inclusion in a youth culture as it is about social exclusion from the dominant 'external' adult culture that surrounds them. Drug consumption is therefore an active expression of what it actually *means* to be a young person.

Young people's drug use as emblematic of unsuccessful socialization

Young people's drug use can be viewed as an emblem of unsuccessful socialization: it demonstrates a lack of successful socialization in appropriate techniques of self-surveillance and self-control. Located on the margins of citizenship, young people's paths through traditional routes to adulthood and full citizenship are seen as blocked if they use drugs. However, as implied above, youth transitions that are intersected by risky or disordered consumption such as drug use are not necessarily blocked. Many, if not most young, people survive the transition and find routes into adulthood.

Nevertheless, while many young people may survive difficult transitions or become resourceful in the face of restructured transitions into adulthood (Roberts 1997), all will have increasing difficulties if their rights as citizens are denied (Dean 1997). Young people are both consumers and citizens or, as Jones and Wallace (1992) contend, young people are 'consumer citizens'. Indeed, through citizenship, young people are endowed with universal rights that are grounded in their social existence. Significantly, these rights are not proportionate to their market value. But when groups of young people 'short circuit' their positions in the cycle of production, reproduction and consumption through drug use, they are seen to lose ground as citizens. Whether or not they are disillusioned with their parents, adults or 'the system', they are viewed as 'disaffected', 'dispossessed' or 'undeserving' youth. While young people's use of drugs extends the notion of consumption into the domains of health, medicine and therapy (Griffin 1997), this use propels them as consuming subjects to the outer boundaries of citizenship.

Young people as consumers of drug services

As noted above, young drug users are often propelled into the health, medicine and therapy domains. In this context, the realm of drug services that intersects these domains is 'qualitatively' different from other realms of health care, not least because of the illegal nature of drug use (see Bennett 1989) and the risks of HIV/AIDS (Rhodes 1994). Furthermore, we see two additional reasons that can be used to explain the qualitative difference between drug services and other health care services. Firstly, there is an in-built and often hidden 'blaming the consumer' approach in most drug treatment regimes. Secondly, treatment consumers tend to experience a contradictory relationship with drug services. But, how does the 'blaming the consumer' approach impact on the young?

Young drug users and the 'blaming the consumer' approach

In other realms of health care, we tend to blame the treatment regimes, service providers, treaters, and so on, if something goes wrong. In the realm of drug service treatment, we blame the patient, client, customer or consumer. We know that young people are constructed and managed by society in a variety of treatment regimes of care and control (Griffin 1997). When young people enter drug treatment regimes, they are constructed by and pressed into a 'drug consumption related' transition. For example, at the same time that the young confront their transition into the adult cycle of production, reproduction and consumption, they are forced to tackle the transition of becoming drug free, which is performed in an atmosphere of treatment, rehabilitation, care, control and surveillance.

Within drug services, young people's successful transition into a drug-free existence is premised upon their learning self-control, stopping their disordered consumption, and mapping out their future goals (i.e. embracing wholeheartedly the cycle of consumption, reproduction and production which aids their transitions into adulthood). Ultimately, treatment success for young people is about 'unblocking' their routes to adulthood and removing any barriers to full citizenship. If young drug users do not succeed in this atmosphere of intervention, they are blamed. Furthermore, being unsuccessful in this way means that these young people are seen as failures in their transition into adulthood and in their attempts to become drug free. But responses from the adult and drug intervention worlds can be a hidden component of drug-related harm for young people; they may experience exclusion in various contexts (i.e. school, peer groups, family, etc.) and, for some, a criminal record (Ashton 1999).

Here drug treatment services can be seen as part and parcel of an interventionist state because these services co-opt community institutions like the family and the educational organizations into a system of repressive control (MacGregor 1995). Whether or not they are successful in their transition into a drug-free state, young drug users who have gone through drug treatment may find that they are viewed as 'damaged goods' and ultimately as 'second-class citizens'. They have dared to consume a risk product (and thus, polluted their once 'healthy bodies'). They have endangered their transition into adulthood and have therefore disowned the right to be 'deserving' citizens.

Young people and their contradictory relationship with drug services

In the above context, it is not surprising that as drug service consumers young people tend to experience contradictory relationships. On the one hand, the young may acknowledge that their drug consumption is problematic. On the other hand, they may also believe that treatment services have nothing to offer them (Fountain et al. 2000). Crome et al. (2000) contend that drug services, in order to be appealing to young people, must aim to attract, engage and retain young people in a service provided by a multi-professional team within a multi-agency partnership. For the young, the therapeutic world of drug services may be viewed as offering 'adult, external' help or facilitating their stopping drugs, but experienced as repressive. The problem is that young drug users are viewed as a special 'high risk' population of drug consumers in need of more intensive interventions than adult drug users (Gilvarry 1998).

Drug services provide young drug users with models of conforming cultures in both statutory and non-statutory settings. But these models tend to impose notions of transitions that privilege blame, victimization or personal deficits vis-à-vis young people's drug consumption. McIntosh and McKeganey (2000) note that a recipe for successful transition into a drug-free life is engagement in non-drug-related activities and relationships. If this is so, young drug users in treatment need to focus on harm reduction, self-surveillance and self-control as service resources aiding successful transitions rather than as forms of repressive control. Given that the young do not always believe in the dangers of certain types of drug consumption, an emphasis on negativity or the risks and dangers of drug use will result in poor prevention strategies (Morgan et al. 1999). Furthermore, it would seem that instilling an awareness of the sociality of treatment (i.e. treatment is a complex social interaction process) among both providers and consumers (Lilley et al. 2000) would make sense. Thus, when treaters attempt to embed models of conforming cultures into drug services, they need to take into account that as a social process, treatment has a particular impact on the young. Those young people who attend services will come with their own sanctions and rituals of drug consumption (Moore 1993). Thus, services need to avoid approaches, which are patronizing, dishonest, and insulting (Teeman et al. 1999). Regrettably, this may be a formidable task, given that drug services appear to continue to employ a pathological model of youth.

Conclusion

In conclusion, we have attempted to show that the problem with discourses on youth consumption and, specifically, discourses on young people's consumption of drugs and drug services, is that these discourses focus on young drug users as being unhealthy, risky consumers and symbols of unsuccessful socialization. These images tend to reinforce a pathological model of youth, stigmatizing young people unnecessarily. Furthermore, this pathological model of youth forms the basis of drug services' responses to young users. While drug services tend to uphold an in-built and often implicit 'blaming the consumer' approach, this has a negative impact on young drug users. Furthermore, young people who are consumers of drug services experience a contradictory relationship with drug services: they experience drug use as problematic but they don't see services as helpful to them.

We hope we have illustrated the limitations of this sort of approach to young people's consumption in the context of drugs and drug services. While discourses on consuming health are important for the young to internalize, we must try to account for the pleasurable aspects of young people's patterns of consumption in our work. Young people's drug consumption should not be viewed moralistically, and not merely as part-and-parcel of many young people's everyday lives, but rather as an active expression of what it actually means to be a young person in an uncertain world. Only when youth and drug researchers achieve their own transition in this respect, and only when research genuinely realizes why young people enjoy drugs, will the drug services provide the young with what they actually need. As citizens of a 'risk' society, young people are constantly confronted by threats to their health and well-being. But in many respects their choice to partake in drugs as a risky form of consumption represents an effort to balance the demands and tensions of an increasingly individualized world. It is therefore absolutely essential that the meanings with which young consumers endow their drug use – and, for that matter, any other form of allegedly 'unhealthy' behaviour – play a pivotal role in the sociological exploration of 'health consumption'.

References

Ashton, M. (1999) 'Between two stools: children, drugs policy and professional practice', in A. Marlow and G. Pearson (eds) *Young People, Drugs and Community Safety*, Lyme Regis: Russell House Publishing Ltd.

Balding, J. (2000) *Young People and Illegal Drugs into 2000*, Exeter: Schools Heath Education Unit.

Beck, U. (1992) *Risk Society: Towards a New Modernity*, London: Sage.

Bennett, G. (ed.) (1989) *Treating Drug Abusers*, London: Tavistock/Routledge.

Berridge, V. (1998) 'AIDS and British Drug Policy', in M. Bloor and F. Wood (eds) *Addictions and Problem Drug Use: Issues in Behaviour, Policy and Practice*, London: Jessica Kingsley.

Blackman, S.J. (1996) 'Has drug culture become an inevitable part of youth culture? A critical assessment of drug education', *Educational Review*, Spring: 131–42.

—— (1997) '"Destructing a giro": a critical and ethnographic study of the youth "underclass"', in R. MacDonald (ed.) *Youth, the 'Underclass' and Social Exclusion*, London: Routledge, pp. 113–29.

Brain, K., Parker, H. and Carnwath, T. (2000) 'Drinking with design: young drinkers as psychoactive consumers', *Drugs: Education, Prevention and Policy*, 7, 1: 5–20.

Brannen, J., Dodd, K., Oakley, A. and Storey, P. (1994) *Young People, Health and Family Life*, Buckingham: Open University Press.

Bunton, R. and Burrows, R. (1995) 'Consumption and health in the "epidemiological" clinic of late modern medicine', in R. Bunton, S. Nettleton and R. Burrows (eds) *The Sociology of Health Promotion*, pp. 206–22.

Burke, K.C., Burke, J.D. Jr, Regier, D.A. and Rae, D.S. (0000) 'Age at the onset of select mental disorders in five community populations', *Archive of General Psychiatry*, 5: 511–18.

Cashmore, E.E. (1984) *No Future: Youth and Society*, London: Heinemann.

Collison, M. (1996) 'In search of the high life: drugs, crime, masculinities and consumption', *British Journal of Criminology*, 36, 3: 428–44.

Crome, I., Christian, J. and Green, C. (2000) 'The development of a unique designated community/drug service for adolescents: policy, prevention and education implications', *Drugs: Education, Prevention and Policy*, 7, 1: 87–108.

Dean, H. (1997) 'Underclassed or undermined?: Young people and social citizenship', in R. MacDonald (ed.) *Youth, the 'Underclass' and Social Exclusion*, London: Routledge, pp. 55–69.

Ensign, J. and Gittelsohn, J. (1998) 'Health and access to care: perspectives of homeless youth in Baltimore City, USA', *Social Science and Medicine*, 47, 12: 2087–99.

Featherstone, M. and Hepworth, M. (1998) 'Ageing, the lifecourse and the sociology of embodiment', in G. Scambler and P. Higgs (eds) *Modernity, Medicine and Heath*, London: Routledge, pp. 147–75.

Fountain, J., Strang, J., Griffith, P., Powis, B. and Gossop, M. (2000) 'Measuring met and unmet needs of drug users: integration of quantitative and qualitative data', *European Addiction Research*, 6, 2: 97–103.

Furlong, A. and Cartmel, F. (1997) *Young People and Social Change*, Buckingham: Open University Press.

Gilvarry, E. (1998) 'Young drug users: early intervention', *Drugs: Education, Prevention and Policy*, 5, 3: 281–92.

Griffin, C. (1997) 'Troubled teens: managing disorders of transition and consumption', *Feminist Review*, 55: 4–21.

Henderson, S. (1999) 'Drugs and culture: the question of gender', in N. South (ed.) *Drugs: Cultures, Controls and Everyday Life*, London: Sage.

Jones, G. (1995) *Leaving Home*, Buckingham: Open University Press.

Jones, G. and Wallace, C. (1992) *Youth, Family and Citizenship*, Buckingham: Open University Press.

Lilley, R., Quirk, A., Rhodes, T. and Stimson, G. (2000) 'Sociality in methadone treatment: understanding methadone treatment and service delivery as a social process', *Drugs: Education, Prevention and Policy*, 7, 2: 163–78.

MacGregor, S. (1995) *Drugs Policy, Community and the City*, London, Middlesex University, School of Sociology and Social Policy Occasional Paper.

—— (1999) 'Medicine, custom or moral fibre: policy responses to drug misuse', in N. South (ed.) *Drugs: Cultures, Controls and Everyday Life*, London: Sage.

McDonald, K. (1999) *Struggles for Subjectivity: Identity, Action and Youth Experience*, Cambridge: Cambridge University Press.

McIntosh, J. and McKeganey, N. (2000) 'The recovery from dependent drug use: addicts' strategies for reducing the risk of relapse', *Drugs: Education, Prevention and Policy*, 7, 2: 179–92.

Measham, F., Aldridge, J. and Parker, H. (2000) *Dancing on Drugs: Risk, Health and Hedonism in the British Club Scene*, London: Free Association Books.

Miles, S. (2000) *Youth Lifestyles in a Changing World*, Buckingham: Open University Press.

Miles, S., Cliff, D. and Burr, V. (1997) ' "Fitting in and sticking out": consumption, consumer meanings and the construction of young people's identities', *Journal of Youth Studies*, 1, 1: 81–96.

Montgomery, S. and Schoon, I. (1997) 'Health and health behaviour', in J. Bynner, E. Ferri and P. Shepherd (eds) *Twenty-Something in the 1990s: Getting On, Getting By, Getting Nowhere*, Aldershot: Ashgate, pp. 77–96.

Moore, D. (1993) 'Social controls, harm minimization and interactive outreach – the public health implications of an ethnography of drug-use', *Australian Journal of Public Health*, 17, 1: 58–67.

Morgan, M., Hibell, B., Andersson, B., Bjarnason, T., Kokkevi, A. and Narusk, A. (1999) 'The ESPAD Study: implications for prevention', *Drugs: Education, Prevention and Policy*, 6, 2: 243–56.

Nava, A. and Nava, O. (1990) 'Discriminating or duped?', *Magazine of Cultural Studies*, 5: 15–21.

Parker, H., Aldridge, J. and Measham, F. (1998) *Illegal Leisure: The Normalization of Adolescent Recreational Drug Use*, London: Routledge.

Plant, M. and Plant, M. (1992) *Risk-Takers: Alcohol, Drugs, Sex and Youth*, London: Routledge.

Rhodes, T. (1994) *Risk Intervention and Change: HIV Prevention and Drug Use*, London Health Education Authority in association with the National AIDS Trust.

Roberts, K. (1995) *Youth Employment in Modern Britain*, Oxford: Oxford University Press.

—— (1997) 'Is there an emerging British underclass? The evidence from youth research', in R. MacDonald (ed.) *Youth, the 'Underclass' and Social Exclusion*, London: Routledge, pp. 39–54.

Rutherford, J. (1997) Introduction, *Soundings*, 6: 112–26.

Smith, D.J. and Rutter, M. (1995) 'Time trends in psychosocial disorders of youth', in M. Rutter and D.J. Smith (eds) *Psychological Disorders in Young People: Time Trends and Their Causes*, Chichester: Wiley.

South, N. and Teeman, D. (1999) 'Young people, drugs and community life: the messages from the research', in A. Marlow and G. Pearson (eds) *Young People, Drugs and Community Safety*, Lyme Regis: Russell House Publishing Ltd.

Teeman, D., South, N. and Henderson, S. (1999) 'Multi-impact drugs prevention in the community', in A. Marlow and G. Pearson (eds) *Young People, Drugs and Community Safety*, Lyme Regis: Russell House Publishing Ltd.

Chapter 11

Consuming men's health

Risk, ritual and ambivalence in men's
lifestyle magazines

Robin Bunton and Paul Crawshaw

Introduction

In recent years *Men's Health* has gained prominence on health promotion and public health agendas. This phenomenon can be attributed to a growing recognition that men experience significant inequalities in terms of health outcomes and is reflected in both the provision and uptake of services. Researchers and practitioners have concluded that men are the 'weaker sex' in terms of health (Sabo and Gordon 1995) and have attributed this to the problem of 'masculinity' as a gender identity as well as to their readiness to participate in 'risky' health behaviours and ignore preventative advice. Poor health among men can thus be seen as the result of attempts to consolidate masculine identities by developing risky lifestyles (Watson 1998). Masculinity, then, can be understood as a key risk factor associated with male experiences of health and illness; not only a risk factor in disease aetiology, but also as a definite barrier to developing consciousness about health and illness (Cameron and Bernades 1998). The emerging concern with men's health is apparent in men's consumption of health care and products and is reflected in consumption sites such as men's lifestyle magazines.

Concern for men's health has been reflected in policies that have attempted to target men as a hard-to-reach group. Interventions have taken many forms, from establishing initiatives to target men in traditionally masculine environments such as public houses and working-men's clubs, to media campaigns that attempt to raise awareness of issues such as testicular cancer. In the UK, for example, increased concern for men's health resulted in the launch by the Department of Health of two websites in 2000 providing information for users and health practitioners addressing men's health issues. Such interventions have largely taken place outside of clinical medicine and are part of the rise of what Armstrong (1983) referred to as 'surveillance medicine'. Men's self-health care reflects a broader strategy of recent Western health care policy to engender enterprising, self-managing citzenships. Men are being encouraged to monitor their own health and behaviours through such practices as checking for testicular cancer and cutting down alcohol intake. Men and women are thus being constructed as self-monitoring and reflexive healthy citizens. 'Looking after yourself' is encapsulated in health care strategies and takes health beyond the hospital walls into other sectors. Health is, as O'Brian notes (1995), increasingly de-differentiated. That is, health now enters all sites of social and cultural reproduction, including sites of consumption, and is not restricted to the 'health sector'. Contemporary marketing of health, in public and private spheres, has resulted in the development of an array of health products and 'lifestyles' to be promoted and sold. Increased availability of healthy products circulates symbols of health and well-being in newer and more pervasive ways. Nowhere is this more prominent than within 'lifestyle' magazines, including those for men, such as *Men's Health*, *GQ* and *FHM*. These texts are constitutive of the commodification of health and reproduce the signs and values given to health products for men. Magazines are products in themselves, consumed in everyday settings, but they are also a means of conveying consumer cultures surrounding health. In line with the well-established women's titles such as *Cosmopolitan*, men's lifestyle magazines provide opportunities for reflexive monitoring of behaviours and practices which serve to construct masculine identities within contemporary consumer cultures. The construction of such identities is often a complex and contradictory process as men struggle to combine masculine coded 'risky' behaviours with a concern with their own health and well-being, which involves restraint and an ascetic approach to the body. Magazine texts can illustrate the 'de-differentiation' of health within contemporary cultures and the construction of readers/consumers of health advice within a complex gendered identity. In consuming such health messages men are subject to contradictory cultural values relating to good citizenship and 'masculinity'. Consumption involves the resolution of conflicts in various ways. In this chapter we examine some of the contradictory valuations of male health and embodiment in one particular men's lifestyle magazine, *FHM*. We suggest that such texts attempt to resolve inherent cultural contradictions by use of irony and somewhat ritualistic responses to these health concerns. A central contradiction is that between the increased emphasis of consumer cultures for men to consume alongside so-called 'production' values that stress self-discipline and regulation or governance of one's behaviour in the name of health. Lifestyle magazines, we argue, illustrate an unresolvable tension between these two values which can only be played out in ritualistic treatments of health messages.

Magazines, consumption and health governance

One consequence of the onset of consumer culture in the second half of the twentieth century was the breakdown of the sectorization of existence associated with modernism, such as the separation of work and play, shopping and leisure and the healthy and the ill in society. This has been paralleled by the weakening of traditional identity boundaries based around relations of production such as class, gender and sexuality and is said to allow degrees of identity choice. Within contemporary consumer cultures, health extends its narrow sectoral focus, becoming a pervasive element of everyday life, identifiable at sites of consumption both alongside and interacting with leisure and work. Within consumer cultures the 'healthy self' is defined not simply by the absence of illness, but also by his ability to participate fully within communities and consume appropriately (Bunton and Burrows 1995; Burrows and Nettleton 1998). Contemporary health status is thus achieved by purchasing the signs of a healthy lifestyle, from low fat spreads to fitness club membership.

Featherstone (1991) has identified a general tendency for consumer cultures to privilege outward appearance in relation to identity and to 'aestheticize' the body. Health discourses become important resources drawn upon by 'the new cultural intermediaries' (Bourdieu 1984), working in advertising and the new cultural industries, and promoting healthy lifestyle and healthy consumer products. Preventative health discourses promoting the avoidance of risk can be marketed within consumer cultures promoting an ethical disciplined, ascetic bodily regulation, seen for example in practices of healthy eating (Lupton 1996; Coveney 2000). Through consumption of health products and messages, health is digested as the duty of the individual. Contemporary citizens are expected to choose healthy lifestyles and exhibit healthy behaviours as a part of the duty of modern citizenship (Petersen and Lupton 1996). A health imperative is communicated through sites of consumption as diverse as the marketing of foods and health-giving products and warnings on tobacco products, to lifestyle advice in magazines such as those that are to be our focus here.

Magazines have been selected here as a vantage point from which to explore concerns relating to men's health within consumer culture. It is argued that these texts allow us to analyse the positioning of the contemporary subject of health discourses and the acquisition of techniques for constructing the healthy self. Reflecting broader shifts in consumption and health noted above, an increasingly educated population is taking a more active role in its own well-being and interest has emerged in easily accessible sources of health information (Cameron and Bernades 1998). As a result, both newspapers and magazines become important information sources, often devoting whole sections to health topics and health research (Yeaton et al. 1990). Extensive research has been conducted into women's magazines and popular representations of femininity (see Winship 1987; McRobbie 1991) and this is becoming an established area of scholarship (McRobbie 1996). By contrast, as Collier notes (1992), men's magazines are under-researched as a phenomenon. Some studies have begun to consider how masculinity is portrayed within magazines and other media sources (see

Vigorito and Curry 1998; Lyons and Willott 1999; Stevenson *et al.* 2000). The depiction of men's health for male audiences, however, is largely under-investigated.

Magazines are an established form of entertainment and source of information with innumerable titles being produced on a weekly, bi-weekly, monthly and quarterly basis. They are aimed at a broad variety of audiences, and range from specialist magazines concerned with particular interests to more general lifestyle magazines. Magazines specifically aimed at women have existed for over a century (Ballaster *et al.* 1991) and, as noted above, their analysis has become an established area of research by feminist scholars keen to decode their depictions of normative femininity. The successful marketing of 'general interest' magazines for men is, however, a relatively new development (Jackson *et al.* 1999) and this is paralleled by a lack of research into their content. Jackson *et al.* (1999) go on to note that until recently magazines for men were either special interest or porno-graphic, with such genres dating back to the 1940s. The emergence of the lifestyle magazine which covers a broad range of issues, including health, yet still typically incorporates what are seen as the traditional male interests often dealt with in 'specialist magazines' (cars, sport, pornography), is much more specifically a late twentieth-century phenomenon.

Research into women's magazines explored how the genre can be understood as a site for the governance of gender and sexuality through the depiction and construction of normative femininity (see Winship 1987; McRobbie 1991). Within the newer 'lifestyle' magazines we see an increasing concern with the governance of health and health behaviours. This concern is in line with contemporary neo-liberal discourses which serve to construct the individual as responsible for the creation of the healthy self. This governance of health within such magazines reflects broader trends within contemporary neo-liberal ideologies which present opportunities for self-actualization with reference to expert discourses (Bunton 1997). Within contemporary health promotion discourses the pursuit of health and the avoidance of risk has increasingly been presented as a moral imperative (Gillick 1984) with the rational individual making informed choices based on established wisdoms. In this way care of the self is constructed as an individual responsibility and the healthy body is increasingly understood as the morally correct and socially acceptable body. The risk-taking body (the smoker, excessive drinker, non-exercising) is increasingly seen as deviant (Thorogood 1992). Lupton has argued that 'the dominant theme of lifestyle risk discourse is the responsibility of the individual to avoid risks for the sake of his or her own health as well as the greater good of society' (Lupton 1993: 429). This has developed to the extent that it has been described as 'healthism' (Crawford 1984). Such neo-liberal strategies construct the individual with specific relationships to the social world and serve to create the hyper-responsible self who will conform to 'distant' expert discourses (Rimke 2000). This process is inextricably linked with the governance of populations as 'health becomes idealized as self-governed lifestyle choice' (Bunton and Burrows 1995: 210). Within consumer culture magazines have come to provide a channel for expert discourses which offer opportunities for the reflexive construction of the self. They also serve to individualize and regulate consumers whose autonomy is decreased by dependence on discourses which have moved from the clinic to the coffee table. Contemporary lifestyle magazines are a key source of health information, with large sections often being dedicated to health advice relating to such areas as diet, fitness, alcohol and sexual health. In this way, such texts come to play a key role in constructing the healthy body. Advice and information on fitness, food and sexual health are combined with leisure, work and personal and social interactions in a complex interplay that allows the construction of the healthy self. Readers are thus positioned as consumers who are presented with a variety of information offering numerous strategies for constructing the healthy self.

This situation becomes more complex when we consider the content of contemporary men's lifestyle magazines which often contain contradictory messages. Alongside articles dispensing advice for healthy living we are presented with images of the risk-taking male, more in keeping with dominant conceptions of the hard, dry, male body pursuing risk in order to affirm masculine status (Jones 1993). The unifying theme of these apparently divergent discourses is their focus upon the male body as the key signifier of masculinity. Healthy, strong, virile male bodies depicting masculine dominance and success in the public sphere are seen alongside the 'risk-taking' body pursuing pleasure through alcohol, drugs and participation in dangerous 'masculine' coded activities, affirming a 'laddish' role within the teenage to thirty-something, male peer group. The male body thus becomes the cultural surface upon which these contradictions are played out. Such discourses attempt to marry the imperatives of health with the masculine need to demonstrate strength and resilience and a capacity to participate in risky practices yet still 'get up the next morning and get on with your career' (cited in Jackson *et al.* 1999). The 'bricoleur' of signs and symbols presented within contemporary men's magazines typifies the diversity of contemporary cultures where we see a complex interplay of messages at the same sites of consumption. As a consequence, such magazines contain an often perplexing mix of information which often appears to be contradictory. This is perhaps unsurprising. Men's health and masculinity enjoy a complex relationship, and recent studies have shown that masculine gender identities are often incongruous with the pursuit of good health (Sabo and Gordon 1995; Watson 2000). It would appear that in order to appeal to their audiences, men's magazines must operate within established discourses of masculinity, much of which can be understood as injurious to health. However, in keeping with the format of lifestyle magazines, men's magazines also deal with the consumption of health and the construction of the healthy self, imposing a process of health governance similar to that found within women's magazines.

Masculinity and representations of the body

As Connell notes (1995), an adequate understanding of the politics of masculinity(ies) within consumer cultures must acknowledge the importance of embodiment.

> True masculinity is almost always thought to proceed from men's bodies. Either the body drives and directs action (e.g. men are naturally more aggressive than women) or the body sets limits to action (e.g. men naturally do not take care of infants).
>
> (Connell 1995: 46)

From this perspective, we can understand the male body as the driving force of masculine identities and behaviours. If masculinity is understood as such a fundamentally embodied identity, it is perhaps unusual that men's health has remained a relatively unproblematized area. We need to consider the nature of dominant masculine values which come to determine the male relationship with the body. It has been suggested that a key element of 'hegemonic' masculinities is a direct rejection of bodily maintenance and self-care in order to assert masculinity. To 'be' or act like a man is to show a lack of concern for care of the self such as dietary regimen or aesthetic enhancement. A concern with bodily welfare is often viewed as un-masculine and associated with homosexuality (Petersen and Lupton 1996). As a result, men are understood as more likely to be 'heroic' risk-takers (Plant and Plant 1992). Recent UK studies have documented that men claim to ignore healthy lifestyle advice and actively seek risk-taking to test and demonstrate the inherent resilience of their bodies (Bunton et al. 1998). There are clear links, therefore, between dominant discourses of masculinity and male attitudes to health and care of the self (Sabo and Gordon 1995; Watson 2000).

The dominant perspective discussed above views masculinity as an identity which is unconcerned with bodily maintenance and actively courts risk, thereby coming under the gaze of health professionals (Sabo and Gordon 1995; Watson 2000). A more complex picture appears, however, when we begin to examine the positioning of male bodies within consumer cultures. Within such discourses we see that increasing concern with 'lifestyle' and the body is often central to these concerns as a key signifier of socially desirable characteristics. Images of the 'good' body are increasingly communicated through sites of consumption, resulting in the construction of the 'desirable' body which increasingly crosses more traditional gender boundaries. As Featherstone (1991: 18) notes, within consumer cultures highly stylized images of the body proliferate and enhanced appearance is a feature of the development of a more marketable self. The quest for the more marketable self is no longer confined to the realm of the feminine. Within cultures, and directed at men, we see the emergence of a vast array of products and behaviours concerned with health, fitness and fighting the ageing process to maintain the 'youthful' body which has become increasingly venerated. This is evident in the new men's lifestyle magazines. These magazines represent a shift from titles traditionally produced for men which dealt with special interests such as cars, fishing or pornography. The new genre is much closer in style to the well-established women's lifestyle magazines whose content is focused on what have often previously been seen as exclusively feminine interests such as health, beauty, fashion and relationships. A glance through any issue of *Arena*, *GQ* or the newer *FHM* or *Loaded* magazines will reveal content relating to these same areas, including advertisements for skin care products and pictures of fashionable clothes or tips on grooming. These magazines represent a shift from the consumption by men of specific activities and interests to a much broader concern with lifestyle and the consumption of identities. '*FHM* Man' is constructed as young(ish), single, successful in work, successful with the opposite sex, fit and active and concerned about his body, yet also knowing how to have a good time with his mates. The focus is much less on specific areas of interest but much more on a general 'maleness' which is distinct from the female but shares many of the same interests. The outcome of this is that such magazines present numerous 'masculinities' for readers to consume and endless possibilities for the reflexive construction of the self. Health is only one part of this diverse content; under the unifying banner of lifestyle, an almost obsessive concern with the body permeates many of the pages of these magazines.

Men's magazines as 'discourses of masculinity'

The study of texts such as magazines is not new to social science and has in recent years become established as a key area of research (Fiske 1991). Traditional analysis has focused upon content and how this is communicated to the reader using fairly deterministic linear models (Shannon and Weaver 1949) which assume an unreflexive audience. Such content analysis is typically concerned with identifying the key themes within texts, aiming to quantify the frequency with which these emerge, often using this as a basis upon which to explore and interpret the messages they are attempting to communicate to their audiences and the key areas such texts describe. As a consequence, however, as Lupton (1992) notes, the conclusions drawn by content analysis are largely limited to the manifest meanings of such texts. Thus, only the surface meanings, such as the main subject area of a newspaper article or the obvious rhetoric employed therein, are discussed in content analysis. Our analysis of men's magazines has attempted to explore the meanings of textual representations and how they come to represent and reproduce dominant understandings of masculinity and health within consumer cultures. Texts are approached as constituent and active elements of cultures, which are part of a process of the construction of dominant discourses. The purpose of such discourse analysis is to understand how social reality is negotiated as part of an ongoing process between texts and the audience. Texts and textual devices are treated as social processes and practices and patterns of discourses are seen as constitutive of reality both reflecting and producing social, political and economic forces (Lyons and Willott 1999). Discourse analysis focuses upon research into the area of contemporary culture and society attempting to document the links between textual and oral communication and their links to society and social change (Lupton 1992). It can therefore serve to highlight the reproduction of ideology and hegemony in such processes, and the links between discourse structures and social interaction in situations. In many ways, magazine texts epitomize contemporary cultural forms. Their eclectic content made up of signs and symbols with often limited textual content and heavy use of images to represent contemporary gendered discourses.

Consuming health, illness and the body in a popular men's magazine

The analysis of magazine texts discussed here is a part of ongoing research on health and magazines. The examples discussed are drawn from a two-year sample (24 issues) of *For Him Magazine* (*FHM*), published in 1998 and 1999, which was analysed using the method of discourse analysis discussed above. *FHM* is typical of the genre of men's lifestyle magazines as it contains content relating to a range of interests, including sport, leisure pursuits, work, women and health. Health is a regular element of this content with at least one article per issue being devoted to it.

A brief glance at any issue of *FHM* (or any issue of other magazines within the genre of men's lifestyle) confirms that it is very concerned with bodies. The pages are dominated by presentations of the female body within the male gaze and typically depicted as soft, open and accessible to men, in a way that is often consistent with depictions of what are seen as 'soft' pornographic images of women that we would find in more specifically 'adult' men's magazines (Moye 1985). Within such contexts women are frequently presented as 'limited beings with a restricted sexual presence subservient to apparently specific masculine desires' (Moye 1985: 45). The male form is also present in *FHM* but is presented in a greater variety of ways than the female. Male bodies range from the hard body, ready for action, the well-groomed and almost feminine body ready to perform in the public sphere, to the risk-taking body undertaking masculine-coded excesses in pursuit of pleasure and the reaffirmation of masculine status. It is this diverse presentation of the male body for consumption by a largely male readership, and its relevance to men's health, which is our concern here. Below we focus on examples of text from this sample to illustrate three concerns: the hard body, the soft body and the ironic body. These will be used to discuss different constructions of 'masculine health'.

Consuming the hard body: 'learn to do this'

This article, taken from the December 1999 issue of *FHM*, presents a lurid example of the depiction of the male 'hard' body as it is presented in men's magazines and reflects constructions of male bodies within traditional gender discourses. Within such discourses the male body is typically presented as hard, dry and invulnerable. The male body is thus constructed as strong and powerful and able to possess space and dominate others. The bodies of the martial arts fighters depicted in this article are used to show the hard body engaging in practices which demonstrate the body's resilience. The courting of risks is culturally coded as masculine within gender discourses. Saltonstall (1993) suggests that men typically understand a fit, healthy body to be one over which they are in control. Martial artists, such as Bruce Lee, are presented in this article as being in complete control of their bodies, exhibiting the traits of 'real' manhood. We hear, for example, how Bruce Lee responded to a serious injury:

> Bruce executed a high kick and broke two of his ribs, pulling a back muscle and damaging a sacral nerve. He was hospitalized and doctors told him he would never kick again. He was back in action inside six months.
>
> (*FHM* December 1999)

We see a reverence for such bodies which are so firmly under control they may even overcome medical discourses. Bodies like these are seen to represent the ideal male body within Western cultures, the Hellenic, muscular body standing for control, rigidity and strength (Bunton *et al.* 1998). Such bodies are perceived as hard, dry, self-contained and subject to discipline, which means that they can always be controlled, in contrast to feminine bodies which are understood to be moist, leaky and flowing (Shildrick 1997). *FHM* man is unlikely to be able to exercise such control over his body and demonstrate such rigidity and strength, but he can admire such bodies as the idealized, Hellenic masculine form and consume such images as he consumes the broader masculinities presented within such magazines. The martial arts fighter thus becomes a metaphor for masculinity through his ability to exercise control over his body. The masculine form is presented as hard and invulnerable and this is in line with dominant perceptions of the male body which does not require maintenance and within which concerns for health and physical well-being are typically understood as unmasculine.

Consuming the soft body: 'Patch me up good woman'

'Patch me up good woman' is the title of a graphically illustrated feature on health that appeared in the July 1998 issue of FHM and picks up some familiar themes of men's magazine treatments of health. The article reproduces some classic gender positioning in relation to health, while simultaneously exploring the male 'softer' body, and giving preventative advice on the way. Although the 'hard' resilient nature of men's bodies is reproduced, the door is opened slightly on potential vulnerabilities. In contrast to the previous example, this story approaches the need for self-care and preventative action. It is far from the openly nurturing tone of health pages in women's magazines. The tenor of the article is captured in the strap-line, 'Don't waste time in doctors' surgeries. Heal yourself with our guide to self-diagnosis.' The advice given – on diarrhoea, throat problems and head pains – is, in many ways, similar to those in health promotion literature and that found in health pages in women's magazines. The style, however, is tailored to deal with male fear of the vulnerable, open and leaky body. The symptoms of ill health are exaggerated to absurd levels and treatments such as a tracheotomy, are shown in a way that challenge the squeamish as does the main picture of the article which shows a young man tearing his chest open as he heroically deals with illness with strength and denial. (The practice of featuring photographs and articles that test for unmanly squeamishness is common in men's magazines such as *Bizarre*.) John Wayne-like, readers are invited to deal with the mere 'flesh wounds' of battle with a stiff jaw, if not lip, and to be diligently sewn up by attendant women. The association of health with vulnerable, softer bodies, is reinforced in the pictures and the text. A section of the text deals with the dangers of Victorian hospitals and their likelihood of making inmates ill. Similarly, the doctor's clinic is described as a domestic space and one that needs to be avoided.

> Along with the matted, sweaty armpits of Fatima Whitbread and the walk-in wardrobe of Russell Grant, the doctor's waiting room must surely rank as one of the most repellent places in the history of mankind. Packed to the rafters with wailing kids, red-faced adolescents, the vile stench of sickly OAPs [Old Age Pensioners] and you, slap bang in the middle of the revolting lot of them, it's no wonder that men are so reluctant to pay the quack a visit.

The article manages to allude to two other threatening 'hybrid' bodies in the above. The threat felt by a woman shot putter whose athletic body somehow precludes her femininity and a portly, camp, male TV personality. The male body and psyche should be shielded from such bodies, as they should also be separated from vulnerable, younger and older bodies, if they are to maintain their autonomous, impervious, controlled, embodied existence. 'Female' treatment settings threaten violation, or pollution, and need to be excluded. The whole of this article, like others, is humerous and demonstrates irony through hyperbole and excess. It explores topics of a potentially delicate nature for men by distancing them from the embarrassment and discomfort that sickness and vulnerability gives them.

Consuming the ironic body: 'The lush drinks himself fit'

Throughout *FHM* magazine, alcohol consumption is used as a cultural signifier of masculinity. This is illustrated by articles such as 'The demon drink' (January 1999) and 'Get me off the booze' (March 1999) and 'The lush drinks himself fit' (July 1999). The latter article is of particular interest here. Alcohol is discussed within such articles in a variety of ways, seen as a recreational activity, a problem, a means of group solidarity, and even a passport to success. The unifying theme is its 'normalization' within masculine discourses and the routinization of its use. Alcohol becomes an important cultural artefact which signifies success in one's social life, being out for a drink with mates and trying to 'pull' women, being able to prove that one can 'take one's drink', yet it is also acknowledged as an object which harbours risks, so one must learn to drink carefully and in a way that allows the consumption of such an important, cultural commodity without causing too much damage to one's body. The masculine pursuit of pleasure must not be compromised by restrictive health conciousness.

> In this tragic modern world of health conciousness and low-fat mediocrity, drinking is often frowned upon by the fitness fanatic. Determined to prove that it is possible to imbibe while maintaining a near perfect level of health, I purchased the necessary ingredients and conducted three separate clinical trials on a warm Sunday afternoon ...
> (FHM, July 1999: 54)

The rest of this article gives nutritional advice for combating the ill effects of alcohol.

In 'The lush drinks himself fit' we see an ironic presentation of how activities can be appropriated as healthy but still allow individuals to participate in one of the key arenas of hegemonic masculinity – the consumption of risk objects. This illustrates the irony and contradiction implicit within the discursive formations of masculinity constructed within such texts. Men must be able to balance their role as productive members of society, participating and dominating in the public sphere. Yet, they must also be able to transgress bodily boundaries in pursuit of hegemonic masculinity which demands risk-taking in order to attain masculine status. Hence men must manage the contradictions of drinking and maintain well-being in such a way as to be able to participate in both spheres. Therefore, the tone of 'The lush drinks himself fit' is undeniably ironic but at the same time relates to the real male experiences of healthy practices as they seek to manage the contradictions inherent within masculine discourses. The discourses of pleasure and transgression are thus appropriated in the construction of the healthy self.

The notion of pleasure has historically been problematic in public health and health promotion discourses where energies have typically been directed into steering populations away from pleasure-seeking behaviours such as drinking, smoking and illegal drug use in the name of promoting well-being as well as increased regulation and social control. Hedonistic pleasure-seeking is warned against within these discourses, which flag up the risks of such behaviours and emphasize the need for moderation in consumption and engagement in 'safer' practices, or even abstinence. However, recent commentators have suggested that the transgression of such boundaries – i.e. an awareness of consuming 'risk' objects such as alcohol, or engaging in risky practices such as unsafe sex – can actually be a part of the pleasure of participation in such activities (Klein 1993). As Klein notes, inherent in the pleasures of smoking can be the awareness that one is consuming such a potentially deadly substance. Transgression can thus be understood as a key component in constructing the healthy self. Williams (1998) suggests that conceptions of health, in particular the perceptions held by the middle classes, continually oscillate between bodily discipline and corporeal trans-gression: modalities which reflect and reproduce fundamental contradictions within Western culture and late capitalism itself. Williams thus proposes that transgression is always an important aspect of the ascetic body and that healthy bodies must always be transgressive. This becomes particularly significant within consumer cultures as pleasures and pleasure-seeking are increasingly commodified. Within such cultures we are incessantly bombarded with images which invite us to indulge desires and endlessly consume. As Williams (1998) notes, we can now even eat to get thinner, or, as *FHM* tells us, we can drink to get fitter. He concludes that this rests on the perpetuation of an unbridgeable gap between the idealized and the real which leads to the ritualistic consumption of diverse products, practices and ideals. Corporeal release is thus an intrinsic element of increasingly embodied consumer narratives. This is epitomized by 'The lush drinks himself fit', which presents a range of pleasure giving commodities in the form of 'healthy' alcoholic drinks which readers can consume in order to engage simultaneously in pleasure-driven transgression and pleasure seeking, presumably within the important masculine cultural arena of the public house or bar, yet still perceive themselves as consuming a healthy commodity. For Williams (1998), the late modern body in consumer cultures continually oscillates precariously between bodily control and corporeal transgression. Health becomes a moral performance which is constrained by the habitus of individuals who must seek to balance discipline and transgression in the pursuit of the healthy self. 'The lush drinks himself fit' constructs this within an appropriate masculine habitus as readers are presented with opportunities to consume objects that are simultaneously risky, yet healthy. In this way health comes to be consumed as an intrinsic element of masculine identities as the 'healthy' male must be able to engage in risky practices which are coded as masculine, yet also maintain a body which is capable of fully participating in society.

Health, rituals and risk

In the above analysis of three texts from men's magazines, we can identify certain differences and tensions within different constructions of men's health that might be indicative of broader tensions in consumer cultures surrounding health. On the one hand, there are constructions of what might be seen as a traditional 'hard' male embodiment that takes 'heroic' risks and distances itself from the 'womanly work' of health and caring. On the other hand, there would appear to be an emergent 'soft' or at least 'softer' body that displays concerns for health and well-being that are in line with mainstream preventative health messages and bear some similarity to the 'health' pages of women's magazines. There are also narratives that ironically embrace the oscillation between the search for bodily control (or governance) and transgression that Williams (1998) highlights as a part of the body in consumer cultures. It is not surprising to find such diversity and tension in magazines. Beatham (1996) has noted that magazines and periodicals are texts designed for temporary and non-fixed readings, and refuse a single authorial voice. Although this style may fit nicely into a 'late-modern' identity formation which is more transitory and fluid (Bunton 1997), such texts may also illustrate fundamental oppositions in the cultural values of Western societies and attempt to resolve or manage them. There would appear to be central underlying tension between the values of production and consumption. Conflict resolution has been studied in anthropology and sociology with reference to rituals, and this approach has recently been drawn upon to analyse the consumption of health.

Analysis of ritual highlights the routine, everyday, ordinariness of conflict resolution. Ritual is frequently seen as functional in binding together social life in the face of inherently conflicting values and goals generated by broader social structures. Rituals allow social actors to display ambivalence, co-existent multiple motivations or dispositions (Turner 1973). Robert Crawford (2000) has recently analysed health promotion as a set ritual practices that reflect the growing importance of consumption values. Drawing upon such notions, he describes how some contemporary forms of health regime place the self-governing citizen at the centre of broader system conflicts between consumption and production. Crawford argues that health promotion shares many properties of the formal ritual, though performed in everyday settings and attempting to bring a sense of order to potentially troublesome conflicts of values. Similarly, David Armstrong (1993), drawing on the work of Mary Douglas (1966), has described the ways that public health hygiene or 'pollution rituals' attempt to deal with 'unruly regions' of existence such as dangerous environments or risky individual behaviour. In such accounts contemporary subjects are conscious of their own health and willing simultaneously to take up rational self-surveillance and self-governance – essential elements of a ritual act that serves a disciplinary social order. The rituals of public health and health promotion may or may not result in better population and health. They do, however, introduce forms of self-reliance and self-governance, even in the face of pressure to behave 'unhealthily'. Health promotion rituals provide individuals with behavioural repertoires for making sense of widely shared conflicts or dilemmas and some major contradictions between the cultural contradictions of capitalism, that is between consumption and production. As Crawford notes:

> Modern capitalism requires both workers and consumers and therefore two fundamentally different behavioural patters, two opposing personality structures, indeed two ethics.
>
> (Crawford 2000: 221)

> Metaphorically homologous with the conflict-generating logic of economic restructuring, Health promotion can be understood as the ritualized displacement of the middle class's anxious ambivalence about discipline and pleasure on to the medicalized body and the language of somatic well-being.
>
> (Crawford 2000: 224)

The polarities that Crawford refers to are similar to those in Western religious traditions. Mellor and Shilling (1997) identify a tension in Western societies within what they describe as the 'Modern Baroque Body'. The rise of European Protestantism, they argue, features as a force that has engendered patterns of sociality based on individual commitment and contract with an embodied self-discipline and asceticism. There is a pervasive, contractual mentality in modern institutions and in forms of self-identity. Yet, simultaneously, we are witnessing the re-emergence of forms of sociality which would appear to signal the exhaustion of the moral basis for contractual society. They refer to the renewed importance of the sensual experience in defining social relationships within modernity. Drawing on the work of

Bataille (1985) and Maffesoli (1996) they suggest a recent tendency towards forms of 'sensual solidarity' and attempts to 're-consecrate the profane', escaping the banal associations of contractual society and seeking newer forms of community and newer forms of embodiment. These opposing forms of embodiment are opposing ethics and disposition towards health risks. We can see such opposing ethics in relation to food, for example, where contemporary dispositions reverberate between constraint and excess (Lupton 1996; Coveney 2000). Such opposing forms of embodiment are apparent in the representation of men's health in magazines and are consumed as contradiction.

In magazine texts we see a variety of dispositions that range from the incitement to ascetic self-regulation (to exercise, eat 'well', develop one's physic and mind) to extremes of aesthetic expression and excess (to indulge in risk-taking and pleasure). Health risk activities are simultaneously celebrated and pilloried. Dispositions towards health are ritually represented and condensed. Pleasure and control are experienced together in these texts. Interdicts to maintain a healthy, hard and efficient body play alongside and make possible the spaces for transgression and pleasure. Eating 'well' allows the opportunity to enjoy the transgressive pleasure of excess. Giving up smoking enables the enjoyment of relapse. Klein (1993) has drawn attention to the continued task of giving up smoking which allows renewed daily pleasures of release from the regimen – the sublime pleasures of transgression. Risk-taking is, as Crawford observes, 'the mirror of health promotion' – doubly charged – 'an effervescence of pleasure and pain – in short, ritualized ambivalence' (p. 228). Health-conscious participants endlessly re-enact their conflicts of 'compliance' and 'resistance', 'restitution' and 'revolt'. Men's health is constructed within similar conflicting narratives which privilege the hard and the soft body simultaneously. The consumption of health in such sites is experienced in a contradictory manner, though perhaps no more so than in other sites of consumption. This contradiction and ambivalence is visible, available and open to analysis in its simultaneity and its irony.

References

Armstrong, D. (1983) *Political Anatomy of the Body: Medical Knowledge in Britain in the Twentieth Century*, Cambridge: Cambridge University Press.

—— (1993) 'Public health spaces and the fabrication of identity', *Sociology*, 27, 3: 393–410.

Ballaster, R., Beetham, M., Frazer, E. and Hebron, S. (1991) *Women's Worlds: Ideology, Femininity and the Woman's Magazine*, London: Macmillan.

Bataille, G. (1985) *Visions of Excess: Selected Writings 1927–1939*, Manchester: Manchester University Press.

Beatham, M. (1996) *A Magazine of Her Own? Domesticity and Desire in the Women's Magazine, 1800–1914*, London: Routledge.

Bourdieu, P. (1984) *Distinction: A Social Critique of the Judgement of Taste*, London: Routledge.

Bunton, R. (1997) 'Popular health, advanced liberalism and Good Housekeeping Magazine', in A. Petersen and R. Bunton (eds) *Foucault, Health and Medicine*, London: Routledge.

Bunton, R. and Burrows, R. (1995) 'Consumption and health in the "epidemiological" clinic of late modern medicine', in R. Bunton, S. Nettleton and R. Burrows (eds) *The Sociology of Health Promotion*, London: Routledge.

Bunton, R., Crawshaw, P. and Green, E. (1998) 'Risk, gender and youthful bodies', unpublished Conference Paper, International Sociological Association XIV World Congress of Sociology, Montreal, August.

Burrows, R. and Nettleton, S. (1997) 'Women's smoking in the employers and managers socio-economic group', *Health Promotion International*, 12, 3, 209–14.

Cameron, E. and Bernades, J. (1998) 'Gender and disadvantage in health: men's health for a change', *Sociology of Health and Illness*, 20, 5: 673–93.

Collier, R. (1992) 'The New Man: fact or fad?', *Achilles Heel*, Winter: 34–8.

Connell, R. (1995) *Masculinities*, Oxford: Polity.

Coveney, J. (2000) *Food, Morals and Meaning: The Pleasure and Anxiety of Eating*, London: Taylor & Francis.

Crawford, R. (1984) 'Healthism and the medicalisation of everyday life', *International Journal of Health Services*, 10, 3: 365–88.

—— (2000) 'The ritual of health promotion', in S. Williams, J. Gabe and M. Calnan (eds) *Health Medicine and Society: Key Theories, Future Agendas*, London: Routledge.

Douglas, M. (1966) *Purity and Danger: An Analysis of Concepts of Pollution and Taboo*, London: Routledge & Kegan Paul.

Featherstone, M. (1991) *Consumer Culture and Postmodernism*, London: Sage.

Fiske, J. (1991) *Introduction to Communication Studies*, London: Routledge.

Gillick, M. (1984) 'Health promotion, jogging and the pursuit of moral life', *Journal of Health Politics, Policy and Law*, 9, 3: 369–87.

Jackson, P., Stevenson, N. and Brooks, K. (1999) 'Making sense of men's lifestyle magazines', *Environment and Planning: Society and Space*, 17: 353–68.

Jones, A. (1993) 'Defending the border: men's bodies and vulnerability', *Cultural Studies from Birmingham*, 2: 77–123.

Klein, R. (1993) *Cigarettes are Sublime*, Durham and London: Duke University Press.

Lupton, D. (1992) 'Discourse analysis: a new methodology for understanding the ideologies of health and illness', *Australian Journal of Public Health*, 16, 2: 145–50.

—— (1993) 'Risk as moral danger; the social and political functions of risk discourse in public health', *International Journal of Health Services*, 23: 425–35.

—— (1996) *Food, the Body and the Self*, London: Sage.

Lyons, A. and Willott, S. (1999) 'From suet pudding to superhero: representations of men's health for women', *Health*, 3, 3: 283–302.

Maffesoli, M. (1996) *The Time of the Tribes*, London: Sage.

McRobbie, A. (1991) *Feminism and Youth Culture: From Jackie to Just Seventeen*, London: Macmillan.

—— (1996) 'More! New sexualities in girls' and women's magazines', in J. Curran, D. Morley and V. Walkerdine (eds) *Cultural Studies and Communications*, London: Arnold.

Mellor, P. and Shilling, C. (1997) *Reforming the Body: Religion, Community and Modernity*, London: Sage.

Metcalf, A. and Humphries, M. (eds) (1985) *The Sexuality of Men*, London: Pluto Press.

Miles, M. (1992) *Carnal Knowing: Female Nakedness and Religious Meaning in the Christian West*, Tunbridge Wells: Burns & Oates.

Moye, A. (1985) 'Pornography', in A. Metcalf and M. Humphries (eds) *The Sexuality of Men*, London: Pluto Press, pp. 44–70.

O'Brian, M. (1995) 'Health and lifestyle: a critical mess? Notes on the dedifferentiation of health', in R. Bunton, S. Nettleton and R. Burrows (eds) *The Sociology of Health Promotion*, New York: Routledge.

Petersen, A. and Bunton, R. (eds) (1997) *Foucault, Health and Medicine*, London: Routledge.

Petersen, A. and Lupton, D. (1996) *The New Public Health: Health and Self in the Age of Risk*, London: Sage.

Plant, M. and Plant, M. (1992) *The Risk Takers*, London: Routledge.

Rimke, H. (2000) 'Governing citizens through self-help literature', *Cultural Studies*, 14, 1: 61–78.

Sabo, D. and Gordon, D. (1995) *Men's Health and Illness: Gender, Power and the Body*, London: Sage.

Saltonstall, R. (1993) 'Healthy bodies, social bodies: men's and women's concepts and practices of health in everyday life', *Social Science and Medicine*, 36, 1: 7–14.

Shannon, C. and Weaver, W. (1949) *The Mathematical Theory of Communication*, Illinois: University of Illinois Press.

Shildrick, M. (1997) *Leaky Bodies and Boundaries: Feminism, Postmodernism and (Bio) Ethics*, London: Routledge.

Stevenson, N., Jackson, P. and Brooks, K. (2000) 'The politics of "new" men's lifestyle magazines', *European Journal of Cultural Studies*, 3, 3: 366–85.

Thorogood, N. (1992) 'What is the relevance of sociology for health promotion?', in R. Bunton and G. MacDonald (eds) *Health Promotion: Disciplines and Diversity*, London: Routledge.

Turner, V.W. (1973) 'Symbols in African ritual', *Science*, 179, 4078 (March): 100–5.

Vigorito, A.J. and Curry, J.T. (1998) 'Marketing masculinity: gender identity and popular magazines', *Sex Roles*, 39, 1/2: 135–52.

Watson, J. (1998) 'Running around like a lunatic: Colin's body and the case of male embodiment', in S. Nettleton and J. Watson (eds) *The Body in Everyday Life*, London: Routledge, pp. 163–79.

—— (2000) *Male Bodies: Health, Culture and Identity*, Buckingham: Open University Press.

Williams, S. (1998) 'Health as a moral performance: ritual, transgression and taboo', *Health*, 2, 4: 435–7.

Winship, J. (1987) *Inside Women's Magazines*, London: Pandora.

Yeaton, W., Smith, D. and Roger, K. (1990) 'Evaluating understandings of popular press reports on health research', *Health Education Quarterly*, 7: 223–34.

Index